SUCCESSFUL PRIVATE PRACTICE IN THE 1990s

A New Guide for the Mental Health Professional

SUCCESSFUL PRIVATE PRACTICE IN THE 1990s

A New Guide for the Mental Health Professional

Joan Kaye Beigel, M.Ed.

Ralph H. Earle, Ph.D.

with

Lynn Fleischman and Ritalinda D'Andrea

BRUNNER/MAZEL, PUBLISHERS • NEW YORK

Library of Congress Cataloging-in-Publication Data
Beigel, Joan Kaye.
    Successful private practice in the 1990s : a new guide for the
mental health professional / Joan Kaye Beigel, Ralph H. Earle with
Lynn Fleischman and Ritalanda D'Andrea.
        p.   cm.
    Includes bibliographical references.
    Includes index.
    ISBN 0-87630-586-9
    1. Psychotherapy—Practice.   I. Earle, Ralph (Ralph H.)
II. Title.
    [DNLM: 1. Mental Health Services.   2. Private Practice.   WM 30
B4225s]
    RC465.5.B45   1990
    616.89'023—dc20
    DNLM/DLC
    for Library of Congress   90-2053
                                                                        CIP

This book contains the advice and experience of expert authorities from many fields.
But the use of a book is not a substitute for legal, accounting, or other professional
services. Consult a competent professional for answers to your specific questions.

Newbridge Book Clubs
For information about our audio products, write us at:
Newbridge Book Clubs, 3000 Cindel Drive, Delran, NJ 08370

Published by
BRUNNER/MAZEL, INC.
19 Union Square West
New York, New York 10003

Manufactured in the United States of America

10 9 8 7 6 5 4 3 2 1

To our "plurking" world—
family, friends, colleagues, and patients/clients

Contents

Acknowledgments

We would like to thank Lynn Fleischman and Ritalinda D'Andrea for their time, patience and creativity in helping to put our ideas into words. We would also like to thank those who contributed their expertise to this book: Connie Bailey; Allan Beigel; Aaron and Mathilda Canter; Tom Courtenay; Margaret DyKinga; Marcus Earle; Steven Engelberg; Sarah Fajardo; Donald Hall; Bob and Jacque Jenson; Jeff Kirkendall; Bonnie McKnight; Marilyn Murray; William Nichols; Frank and Sue Parks; Henry and Diane Reuss; Carolyn Robinson; Harry Saslow; Robert Schwebel; Pearl Selwyn; David Spire; Jeff Stull; John (Matt) Thomas; George Vroom; George Watkins; Jane White; Karen Wiese; Brady Wilson.

Indeed, it is a privilege to receive permission to adapt or directly quote the copyrighted work of other authors. We are pleased to credit the following sources in order of their appearance:

Adaptations from R. F. Warmke, G. D. Palmer and C. A. Nolan (1976). *Marketing in Action* (eighth ed.), pp. 374–377. Adapted with permission from South-Western Publishing Co., Cincinnati, OH.

Quotations from R. Fisher and W. Ury (B. Patton [Ed.]) (1983). *Getting to Yes: Negotiating Agreement Without Giving In.* Reprinted with permission from Houghton Mifflin, New York.

Adaptations from J. Adams (January/February, 1987). The alphabet soup. *The Family Therapy Networker*, p. 24. Reprinted by permission of *The Family Therapy Networker*, 7703 13th Street, N.W., Washington, DC 20012.

Adaptations from R. D'Andrea (April/May, 1988). Health plan alphabet soup: A glossary of terms. *Tucson Magazine*, p. 77. Adapted with permission from *Tucson Magazine*.

Adaptations and quotations from J. Adams (January/February, 1987). A brave new world for private practice. *The Family Therapy Networker*, pp. 20, 21, 25. Reprinted with permission from *The Family Therapy Networker*.

Adaptations from D. Minar (1987). Business Start-Ups: The Professional's Guide to Tax and Financial Strategies. Reprinted with permission from Prentice-Hall, Englewood Cliffs, NJ.

Adaptations from A. D. Farrell (1989). Impact of computers on professional practice: A survey of current practices and attitudes. *Professional Psychology: Research and Practice, 20,* pp. 176, 177. Reprinted with permission from the American Psychological Association, Washington, DC.

Adaptations and quotations from B. McKnight (Fall, 1988). Tips on the promotion of job satisfaction. *Interchange.* Reprinted with permission of Bonnie McKnight, Payroll Tax Control Corporation, 10801 National Boulevard, Los Angeles, CA 90064.

Adaptations and quotations from Ridgewood Financial Institute, Inc. (1984). *Psychotherapy Finances Guide to Private Practice,* Section 3, pp. 2, 4; Section 6, pp. 1–4. Reprinted with permission from Ridgewood Financial Institute, Inc., Hawthorne, NJ.

Adaptations and quotations from S. Engelberg and J. Symansky (March/April, 1989). Ethics and the law. *The Family Therapy Networker,* pp. 30, 31. Reprinted with permission from *The Family Therapy Networker.*

Quotations from American Association for Marriage and Family Therapy (1988). Witness pointers. *AAMFT Legal Consultation Plan Newsletter, III* (3), pp. 3–5. Reprinted with permission from the American Association for Marriage and Family Therapy.

In addition, we could not have realized this book were it not for the participation and feedback of our workshop participants across the country. Finally, we would like to thank our families for their support, conversation, ideas, and encouragement for a far longer time than it has taken to get this book out.

Introduction

Around every corner in the mental health world these days is someone more than willing to predict the imminent demise of private practice. Nicholas Cummings, Ph.D., past president of the American Psychological Association, has stated that the next decade will see the elimination of 50 percent of those now practicing as independent/solo practitioners [Adams, 1987]. Others have estimated that 80 to 85 percent of therapy will be provided through Health Maintenance Organizations (HMOs), Preferred Provider Organizations (PPOs), Employee Assistance Programs (EAPs), and other health care organizations of this sort.*

Changes in delivery systems portend other changes as well. Joan** thinks that our health care system will continue to grow more stratified, resulting in a system similar to that in England: nationalized, social health care with a small number of private doctors (the "Harley Street" doctors) for the very few who can afford them. The U.S. system may have more tiers—private care, private care with insurance reimbursement, semiprivate care through HMOs, PPOs, and so on, nationalized care for the indigent, and little to no care for the "notch" group (that is, those who do not qualify for indigent care but cannot afford or are not eligible for other forms of care)—but the effects of the system will be similar: the number

---

*Also see Definition of Terms in Chapter 5, pp. 99-108.
**In keeping with the conversational, "real world" stance we hope to convey in this book, we speak in the first person frequently. This is not a problem in the plural. To avoid confusion about who is speaking in the singular, however, we have chosen to use the third person ("Joan," "Ralph"). The use of "I" is restricted to direct quotes set off with quotation marks in places where the speaker's identity is clear. The style of this book is deliberately informal and non-academic, in keeping with our focus on business practice.

of therapists able to be supported in private practice under this system will be greatly diminished.

Various reasons have been given to support these claims: the growth of "alphabet soup" organizations (HMOs, PPOs, EAPs, etc.) designed to contain costs, the rising costs associated with private practice (especially malpractice or professional liability insurance), rising fee schedules that some feel will price private practitioners out of the market, and the sheer proliferation of mental health practitioners with varying degrees and kinds of professional training and certification. Redefinition of therapy itself, especially the increasing emphasis on brief therapy, has also contributed to these predictions. Why then this book, if private practice, now on the "endangered species list" according to the prognosticators, is destined for extinction in the near future?

We believe, in spite of dire warnings, that private practice is here to stay. In fact, our prediction is that the 1990s will represent exciting opportunities in private practice not available to us before. These opportunities will not be restricted to any traditional group of practitioners (for example, psychiatrists or psychologists). But there is one catch: the opportunities will most likely be there for THOSE WHO ARE WILLING TO CONCEIVE CREATIVELY OF THEMSELVES AS BOTH THERAPISTS AND BUSINESSPEOPLE. Those in private practice will need to accept the fact that what they do is both a service and a business.

Many, if not most, therapists, however, have a difficult time accepting this premise. If we were to ask most therapists, including those in private practice, if they offer an important "product"—namely, therapy—they would first balk at using that "ugly" word "product" and then answer "yes" to the question. Often these same therapists, however, will contradict their own assessment of therapy's worth by refusing to take seriously the business of providing it.

We can explain some of this antipathy by looking back at what appealed to us about practicing therapy in the first place. Although most of us became therapists from mixed motives, an important one for many of us was altruism, perhaps in direct contradiction to our image of the "hustler/bad guy" businessperson who, instead of helping people, exploits them.

We felt a sense of pride in our motives ("I'm not doing this for the money") and of relief in our actions ("I won't have to practice the dog-eat-dog survival tactics required by the business world").

In other words, we didn't become therapists in order to be businesspeople. What we neglected to examine, however, was the accuracy of what we thought was necessary for businesspeople to do to survive and succeed. One of the premises of this book is that, if you really believe in the value of therapy in the private practice setting, doing the "business" of therapy does not have to be odious nor conducted according to a set of values different from the ones you follow in the practice of therapy, or in your personal life.

This is a book about private practice as a *lifestyle*. It is about seeing what you do—the therapy and the business—as a whole. It is about strategies for success that involve knowing who you are and "capitalizing" on that knowledge.

What this book is *not* is a how-to manual in the traditional sense. It will not tell you what color to paint the walls of your office, whether or not to run an ad in the yellow pages, nor what the best business structure for a private practice is. What it will do, we hope, is present you with a way of thinking about yourself and your practice so that you can answer these questions for yourself.

We are also not trying to say that every therapist is suited for private practice. Part I, on Personal Identity, will help you assess what kind of person you are. We think that making a private practice work takes a particular kind of person—but most people have some aspect of their personalities that, if capitalized upon, can be used to create, build, and maintain a business. Unless there is a side of you that likes to get out (that is, to meet people, to put yourself in different situations and look at them from innovative angles) and create new avenues for your practice, to make things happen, then private practice is probably not the ideal arena for you.

Remember, however, that not all private practices are alike. You may not be the type of person who wants to get out enough to make a solo practice work; practicing with a person who thrives on practice-building to the point of generating enough referrals for both of you (while you take primary responsibility for some other aspect of the practice) or practicing as part of a group may be the perfect arrangement for you.

Remember, too, that life stage will interact with personality. Someone in his or her twenties, recently graduated from school, may not be in the best position to start a private practice. This person would need to possess extraordinary practice-building skills to succeed in establishing a private practice. What would be required for success at this stage might not fit this particular person's personality. This same person, however, in his or her thirties or forties may have established enough connections in the community to succeed with a more moderate level of practice-building activities more congruent with his or her personality. Some other people in their fifties and sixties may have established so great a reputation that only minimal practice-building activities would be necessary; others in this age group might want to establish only a small, part-time practice to supplement retirement income from other sources.

Finally, ideas and beliefs about success and changes in these ideas over time, in addition to personality and life stage, will influence a person's ability to develop a *successful* private practice. Your definition of what it means to be successful will influence the amount and kind of practice-building you will need to do.

It is our thinking, borne out in our workshop experiences over the last several years, that most therapists have a practice-building side to themselves. They simply have not tapped into it because they have not developed a model for building a business based on their own identities and lifestyles. It is not because they don't want to, but rather because no one has taught them how to do it! So, while this book is not a traditional how-to book, it is a training book, or **retraining** book, to help you think about the business of private practice in a way you may not have thought of it before.

In this sense the book is participatory. Throughout the book you will find exercises to help you assess how best to create, build, and maintain your private practice. The questions are open-ended; there are no right or wrong answers, no scores to tally up your chances of succeeding in private practice. The importance of any of these exercises or sample forms we provide is determined by their usefulness to you. To this end, we have also tried to avoid being overly directive. We talk a lot about our own experiences, not because we want to say "this is the one and only right way," but because we want you to see how what we do is based on who we are and to begin thinking about what you can do based on who *you* are.

At times, we also make "global" statements like "therapists are this" or "therapists need to do this"; these statements represent our opinions based on responses of hundreds of workshop participants and others with whom we have discussed our ideas. Our hope is that this structure will encourage you to respond with, "I think this way," or "In my experience, this works, but that doesn't." Periodically, we will include excerpts or actual dialogue from our workshops. These excerpts, called "Listening In," are designed to let you experience directly how other therapists have responded to the questions.

The words *private practice* are themselves a misnomer. If you literally stay private in what you are doing—you do not tell anyone, your clients* do not tell anyone—soon you will have no practice about which to stay private. We have all heard the injunction against starting too many sentences with "I"; it is not "nice" to talk about yourself. Beyond nice, the training of therapists, while not so discouraging as past warnings against revealing personal information to a client, certainly has not gone to the other extreme of "go ahead and talk all you want about yourself." (Nor do we think it should.) The effect of this training, however, is that we are uncomfortable revealing ourselves to clients—yet clients represent one of our primary sources of referrals.

On a social level, some taboos about talking about what we do remain in a culture that still operates within a "sickness" model of therapy. We therefore recognize that some people may be uncomfortable if we talk about what we do; again, the

---

*We have chosen to use the terms *client* and *patient* interchangeably to emphasize the applicability of the ideas presented here to all providers of mental health services.

effect is to render us hesitant to communicate with those who could provide referrals.

All of these factors conspire to keep us from doing the one thing we need to do to succeed in private practice: go public. *If you are not able to share what it is you do, who is going to do it?*

To keep this point clearly in focus throughout this book, hereafter we use the term *independent practice* rather than *private practice.* And because most therapists are not trained to "go public," the largest portion of this book, Part II on Public Identity, is devoted to helping you to devise ways to market yourself and your practice effectively. Chapter 2 discusses some of the resistances you may have toward marketing yourself and provides a model for cooperation rather than competition. The chapter closes with a discussion of ideas about success and how they influence practice-building. Chapter 3 outlines our "formula" for success (which is far from formulaic!) and suggests ways to develop an independent practice lifestyle. Chapter 4 explains exactly how to develop a marketing plan to help you build your practice. We close the chapter with a discussion of the relationship between specializing in a particular aspect of mental health practice and marketing your practice. Finally, Chapter 5 examines various types of large health care organizations, detailing the many opportunities for affiliation that these organizations present to the independent practitioner who wants to remain independent.

The principles and strategies we outline in this book are applicable to all therapists: psychologists, marital and family therapists, social workers, counselors, psychiatric nurses, psychiatrists, pastoral counselors, and so on. One of the points we emphasize is that therapists need to develop both their professional and business effectiveness, and that effectiveness in these areas is not necessarily a function of the academic degree a person has. For example, for years people told Joan, "You'll never make it in independent practice; the only people who make it in independent practice have M.D. or Ph.D. behind their names and can sign for insurance and have other doctors referring to them." This book will show you that this

statement is not true. M.D.s and Ph.Ds are not always successful in independent practice; conversely, we know many
M.A.s, M.Eds and M.S.Ws who arc.

To complement the emphasis on marketing effectiveness in
Part II, Part III on Business and Professional Identity deals
with developing business and professional effectiveness and
discusses issues you need to consider in order to run your
independent practice as a successful small business. Chapter 6
discusses the pros and cons of various types (group, solo) and
legal structures of independent practice. Chapter 7 helps you
determine the physical characteristics of your office (location,
design, furnishings, and so on) that will best reflect the kind of
practice you want. We raise some issues that you as an employer of support personnel need to consider. In this chapter,
we also discuss issues of setting and collecting fees (including
third-party reimbursement) and suggest practices that make
these tasks easier and less traumatic for both therapist and
patient. Finally, we provide some guidelines for your business
and personal financial planning. The first part of Chapter 8
discusses three legal issues—confidentiality, dual relationships, and negligence—which should be of increasing concern
to all mental health practitioners because of the proliferation
of ligation in these areas in recent years. The second part of the
chapter deals with strategies you can use to help protect yourself against legal liability.

Again—we cannot emphasize this point enough—our purpose is not to tell you how to do it, but rather to suggest new
ways of thinking that will allow you to create, or re-create,
yourself as a functioning, energized human being. In this particular reference, developing a successful independent practice in mental health services will be part of this larger identity. However, the principles we discuss can be applied to any
number of independent ventures. Our business is not different
from any other business—except that we must have moral
values that extend beyond the bottom line. If this book helps
you to define both your values and goals and incorporate them
into the creation, growth, and maintenance of your independent practice, then we will have done our job.

PART I
Personal Identity

1/
"Insure Today with Walter Kaye": Define Yourself to Define Your Practice

Bill and Denise* are licensed clinical psychologists in their early thirties. They are business and marital partners. They began their independent practice two years ago and gradually evolved a schedule that meets their personal and professional needs. Each sees 15 clients a week, runs one group, and devotes five to 10 hours per week to building the practice, eight hours a week to record-keeping, and the rest of the time to reading, research, and other professional development. Their primary motivation for entering independent practice was control of their time and the opportunity to work together. They consciously developed a rigid 40 hours per week structure, maintain it, and thrive in it.

Crystal, a psychiatric social worker, left a full-time position at a residential facility after 15 years. At 55, she wants to continue practice but equally wants to pursue her interest in anthropology. She sees 10 patients per week and earns just enough to meet her financial needs. She schedules her appointments on Mondays and Thursdays only and spends the rest of the week at a local college taking classes and reading. She defines herself as quite successful.

Brian is a psychiatrist who holds appointments at a major teaching hospital and a private residential facility and is in

---

* The sketches of therapists we present are composites based on descriptions given to us by workshop participants and others. The names are fictitious.

solo independent practice. His schedule and client load vary, and his teaching, consulting, and therapeutic duties are organized by his very efficient secretary. His earnings are consistently in the six-figure range, and at 60, he describes himself as more fulfilled and enthusiastic than at any other point in his life.

Ronnie, 45, is a marital and family therapist whose patient load fluctuates from three to 20 patient-hours per week. She also teaches at all three universities in her city. Most of her patients are students, former students, their families, and their referrals. Her practice is motivated less by financial requirements and more by the opportunity to work with an interesting clientele.

These therapists lead different lives, but lives of their own design. This freedom constitutes one of the main motivations for going into independent practice. They also define themselves as successful, though their definitions obviously vary. The common thread is *choice.* Their professional and personal identities align. Their personalities, the styles of the therapy they practice, and the characters of their businesses are congruent.

To be successful in independent practice, you need to know and understand your own personality and motivations, not because there is any one personality type required—though certain traits will be helpful—but so that you can consciously choose a business strategy that will allow you to stay in business, resist burnout, and get what you want from the business.

THE HELPER AND THE ENTREPRENEUR

How do you develop that congruence between self and practice? At this point in our workshops we usually ask participants to talk about their work roles. The independent practitioner lives at least two major roles: helper and entrepreneur.

What are the stereotypic traits associated with success in each role?

Compare the traits you associate with each role. Table 1 indicates a composite sample of what workshop participants have listed. The problem is obvious: these two roles are mutually exclusive—and equally unrealistic. Adhering to these stereotypes, while trying to resolve the conflicts inherent in them, is impossible and leads to the failure of many practices and to severe burnout among many practitioners. Belief in these stereotypes is one reason therapists have trouble with areas of their businesses such as public speaking, setting fees, advertising, or talking about what they do. Frequently, people in independent practice need permission to make money.

Both of us have been accused of being hustlers—the quintessential entrepreneurial bad guy—on the basis of this helper/entrepreneur dichotomy. In his second year of family therapy practice with a group in Scottsdale, Arizona, Ralph received an envelope from the Board of Psychologist Examiners. This is not the kind of mail a therapist wants to receive under any circumstances, but certainly not when he or she is new in town and just beginning a practice. Inside the envelope was a letter that a Phoenix man had sent to the State Board, which stated that Dr. Earle was a hustler and documented his unhap-

TABLE 1

Helper	Entrepreneur
receptive	aggressive
objective	persuasive
process-directed	product-directed
altruistic	materialistic
female	male
yin	yang
people-centered	market-centered
educated	street-wise
introverted	extroverted
noble poor	ignoble rich
ethical	unscrupulous
Bambi	Jaws

piness with Ralph's behavior. The Board wanted Ralph to let them know what had happened from his point of view. He replied, and then they sent a letter to the man which indicated that what Ralph had done was standard operating procedure and not a problem. Some of Ralph's friends told him, "He was really giving you a compliment."

Joan has also heard people say, "She's too aggressive, too assertive, she has the New York personality. She's hustling, doing this and that." Here is what Joan says about her background:

I often tell workshop audiences that soon after I popped out of the uterus, I was taught to say "Insure today with Walter Kaye" (my father who owns a large insurance business). I was taught to be charming and interesting to anyone who came along, so no one really frightens me; there is no one to whom I can't say, "Hello, how are you?" etc. I decided I was not going to be in the business world. I wanted to deliver a service, so I decided I would deliver a service called counseling. The two things are not separate in my life.

There is no single right way to do therapy; we choose an approach or some mixture of approaches based on context: our own personality, our training and experience, the patient's personality, and our assessment of the problem at a particular time. There is no single right way to conduct business; we choose activities and strategies based on context: our own personality, our training and experience, our market, and our goal at a particular time. Notice that training and experience appear in both lists. When Ralph has had therapists join him in his group practice, they often say, "We're well trained in [whatever style of therapy], or at least feel most comfortable there." There is never any mention of training in the business of independent practice. Joan was surprised to be asked to do a workshop on independent practice for psychiatrists at her local university medical school. She realized that psychiatrists are taught to work at a distance, and in school they learn all the right techniques, but techniques alone. Many of the people who attend our workshops are very comfortable with the kind of therapy they do because they are well trained. They are not comfortable with the idea of running a business because they have received no training. In our opinion, it requires more than just therapeutic technique to make a business successful, whether in an office behind closed doors or in public.

THE INDEPENDENT PRACTICE "PERSONALITY"

We usually ask our workshop participants to suggest qualities or characteristics, based on their experience, that they think are important in independent practice. Roughly one-half of the people in the workshops are full-time private practitioners; the other half are part-time or thinking about starting a practice. Here is an excerpt from one of our discussions:

Listening In

(*Note*: We always ask participants to state their names and describe their specialties, affiliations, and so on when they first stand up in the workshops. An enormous amount of networking thus takes place. We do not use names in the dialogues excerpted in this book.)

Ralph (R): What qualities do you think are important for somebody in independent practice?
Participant (P): Hungry.
R: Hungry? Motivation—okay. That's a good word.
P: You have to enjoy making decisions.
R: That's great. The enjoyment of decisions. I told you already that for me independent practice is a comfortable home. I've worked in other arenas—on staff, executive director of a counseling center, the university—but independent practice is clearly the place because of the autonomy in making decisions. But making decisions for some people is tough, and if you're going to be in independent practice,

those decisions are going to come up a lot. You can't avoid them and still build a thriving practice.

P: You have to like people.

R: I do believe that's more important in independent practice. As a therapist, of course, liking people is important in any setting. I'm referring more now to the business, practice-building side, for which you may not be responsible in other settings. If you worked in these settings, you wouldn't necessarily need to like people to the extent that independent practice requires.

P: One of the things I like is that I can make things up as I go along.

R: For example, what kinds of things?

P: I like making up workshops and thinking up ways to make new contacts.

R: One of the exciting things for me about independent practice is that it takes a great deal of creativity. I am always looking for ways to improve my practice. Independent practice takes creativity plus. I have a lot of different needs to be satisfied. Independent practice provides that kind of relief. I like to go and build. When I was very young, I sold different products—vacuum cleaners, cookies. Independent practice is selling, too, even though you don't have a tangible product you store in a warehouse or inventory at the end of the month. You can be an excellent therapist, but when you start out by hanging a shingle, competency itself is not going to build an independent practice unless you have a major reputation in a given geographic or specialty area. I like to build; I like to do therapy; I like to be able to get out and help a practice to get larger so it fits that side of my needs. What are some other personality characteristics?

P: I think the ability to organize is important.

R: Yes, efficiency. I see that as a key area in independent practice. I have a group; Joan has a large group. I handle a lot of administrative details, but I don't make money by administering. I don't get paid for doing that, and it's not the part I enjoy the most. When I'm on the clock, the patient's needs come first. When I'm off that clock, then

I'd rather be playing golf or be with my family or doing something else. I tend to sandwich a lot in between a very, very short period of time so that I'm not designating two to three hours a day on administrative details that don't produce income. I've noticed that many of the people with whom we've consulted spend a tremendous amount of time obsessing about the business side. I don't think we get paid for being depressed or worrying about why we're not seeing more people. (If we could market that, some of us would do well.) It hurts the business.

When I'm not seeing people, I do administrative work; then the rest of the time is out of the office, not in the office. At the office, all we're going to run into is ourselves and other therapists; we can't go around in the building trying to bring in new clients. I strongly suggest filling your time. Suppose you're starting a practice and you want to work 35 or 45 hours a week. (I tend to work many hours when I'm in town, but I also travel a lot, spending some of that time vacationing, so there's a balance.) If you have 25 patient-hours and your practice isn't as full as you'd like it to be, then those other 10 or 20 hours need to be filled doing specific activities that might be productive in filling that practice. Get out and start meeting more people instead of staying in the office and worrying about it. What other personality characteristics have you thought of?

P: Nobody has mentioned money yet. You really have to be willing to ask for payment and expect it.

R: Right. That's the bottom line. If we have 50 hours of patients but they don't pay . . . well, that's going to be a problem.

P: One of the things I've noticed in independent practice is that my time is my own, in a sense. It's very different from when I was on staff; you have to like being in charge in a way that is not asked for, nor wanted, in a staff setting.

R: There are two related issues here. One involves the use of your own time; no one is telling you what to do, which means you have the freedom to do what you want and the responsibility to do what needs to be done, from both therapeutic and practice-building perspectives. The other issue relates to being in charge of others. How you feel about this issue will influence the way you structure your independent practice. I don't particularly like to be in charge of others, and I don't want to control the people around me. Thus, my practice is arranged so that everyone has a great deal of autonomy. At the same time, it's my responsibility to make sure the practice as a whole functions well. I have to be willing to take charge when it's needed for the good of the group.

We think there are other personality characteristics that contribute to success in independent practice. Creating an independent practice in the first place takes confidence; confidence is also required to do what you need to do to build the practice, all of which is going to involve risk and the unknown. If you are not confident about both your therapeutic and business abilities, you will have a difficult time succeeding in independent practice. One way you can confront your anxiety is by attending workshops or seminars that deal with business issues. (You may already be confronting your anxiety by reading this book!) Another way is to find someone else in your field in your locality whom you think is successful and buy supervision time from him or her.

Many of these business anxiety issues are therapy issues. If you are not allowed to be successful, you are not allowed to earn money. Joan, for example, has recognized that, because she came from a "comfortable" family, she thought she had to prove how hard working she was. Her office and her personal appearance reflected this no-nonsense approach, which was really a difficulty in accepting herself as the professional she is. Over the last few years, however, Joan has upgraded her office from second-hand furniture to new, professional furniture with pizzazz. She is also dressing in a manner that is professional and appropriately stylish. She feels she is finally "growing into [her] professional being on a personal level." It is important to work through anxiety in an effort to align this personal and professional identity; otherwise, you may do everything *right*, at least to outward appearances, but you will make yourself so nervous and tense, you will wind up sick—and so will your practice.

Here we want to raise a key concept—the notion of appropriateness—to which we will return in greater detail in Chapter 3. We believe that a therapist in independent practice must develop a keen sense of what is appropriate, whether it be in behavior, therapeutic practice, dress, community image, or office image. Joan's previous personal image as evidenced in her dress reflected anxiety about success, about being a professional. To swing to the opposite extreme, however—that is, to dress in an outlandish manner or in a way that is sexually provocative or overly casual (based on the norms for your community and clientele)—is counterproductive to independent practice. The same can be said about extremes in any of these other categories.

Flexibility and availability are also key traits that often go together for independent practitioners. It is difficult today to be in independent practice and not be on 24-hour call. This does not mean that you have to make yourself available to all patients 24 hours a day, seven days a week, 52 weeks a year. It does mean, however, that you have some system in place to handle emergencies; it means you arrange with a colleague to cover for you if you want to be free of responsibility for a time; it means you may have to see a family for the first time late at night, early in the morning, or with very little warning. Joan says,

I tell my clients when they see me the first time, I'm available 24 hours a day except when I'm out of town, and occasionally, even when I leave town, I'll give my number to certain clients whom I believe to be more likely to get into trouble. Just knowing they can reach me if they need to is enough to make them feel okay, and they rarely call. If you conduct your practice appropriately, you receive fewer and fewer emergency calls. I also tell them I am at my therapeutic best between seven in the morning and eight-thirty at night. If they feel a crisis brewing, call then. I tell them I will talk to them at three-thirty in the morning, but I might not be worth much. I also don't give my home number out because I've always had kids around the house. The children take messages, but you never know where a message is. I tell clients to call my answering service. The service calls me, and I call the service frequently.

I also do not charge for emergency phone calls (as distinguished from arranged phone consultation, for example, if a client goes away for a few weeks but wants to conduct his or her regular session by phone). But one client asked me why our regular face-to-face sessions were sometimes 40 minutes long instead of the standard 50 minutes. I explained to her that the shorter sessions were still therapeutically effective, and I reminded her that we had spent two and one-half hours on an emergency phone call the week before when I was out of town, for which I did not charge. I generally give 40-minute sessions to her because I know that when I'm out of town, our emergency phone sessions will be extra-lengthy. I should have told her up front that I feel cheap about charging for phone calls.

For Joan, the answer to emergency or short-notice calls is not to say "No" but to say "Yes" collectively. Some of her colleagues, when asked to see emergency patients, will say, "No, I'm busy," and give the caller three other names to try. Joan's group tries not to do this. The therapist who takes the call will ask what the issue is, what the caller wants, and will make sure that someone sees the caller. On those occasions when everyone in her office is busy, the person taking the call contacts other therapists in the community whom she or he trusts until someone is found to take the patient.

We have to determine individually the level of our flexibility. Ralph points out that in his group practice he is the one who tends to keep the bizarre hours.

I received a call one day from a minister who, with his wife, was doing a marriage enrichment program that evening at a church. They ended up with 95 couples and were overwhelmed; they wanted to know if I could help. This was the last day I was going to be in town for a while, and I was seeing patients until 6 that evening, but I said I would do it. I like to "strike while the iron is hot," both in terms of prevention of later problems for those people attending the program and as a response to a particular person with a need (who is also more likely to become a referral source in the future) as opposed to saying, "I see patients from 7 to 6 and I'll be too tired."

There are, however, limits to all of us. The balance for me is to try to do those activities that make most sense for me when they become available. For someone else, who may even have the same idea about balance, the manifestations of that may be quite different. I think in terms of a family therapist working with our "family." I have great respect for the way each member of our group lives out his or her value system. We have some people who do not start before 8 in the morning. I start seeing patients between 6:15 and 7, and we have groups that start at 7. Some of the people who start later, work later into the evening. It's a matter of finding out what's comfortable in your value system, based on where you are in your life stage, what relationship you want with your family and friends, and what you hope to accomplish.

What are the personality traits and characteristics necessary to succeed in independent practice? You have read some of our ideas and those of other therapists, but the most pertinent answer to this question from your viewpoint lies with you. The design of your practice, if it is to succeed, will follow the same formula that your therapeutic style follows: the style must reflect your values, beliefs, personality, and goals.

The therapeutic community is expert in defining these areas. The challenge is in shaping the relationship between you and your business. If we were helping clients-in-relationship, step one might be to administer personality tests to them. Not a bad idea in this relationship. Depending on your preferences and prejudices, you might refer to your own scores on the MMPI, the Myers-Briggs, the Rorschach, or on Performax's Personal Profile System. Your clinical profile is not important here. Rather the information will indicate some stylistic traits. Remember that there is no one way or one personality style or one belief system that equals success in independent practice. You want to gather information about yourself and shape the practice accordingly. For example, scoring high on the Introversion Scale on the Myers-Briggs does not mean that you cannot market yourself or even that the marketing will be difficult. However, you might find that your best marketing will come from referrals rather than by offering seminars.

We tailored the following questionnaire to help you place yourself and your business in a healthy relationship. After you have finished reading this book, we ask you to retake the Self-Assessment and the Success (Chapter 3) Questionnaires in light of the new ideas presented in the book. These questionnaires are therefore repeated in Appendix I.

SELF-ASSESSMENT

1. List two goals in each of the following categories:

    Personal _____

    _____

    Significant Others _____

    _____

    Professional _____

    _____

    Spiritual _____

    _____

    Humanitarian _____

    _____

    Other _____

    _____

2. List two techniques you are currently using to accomplish these goals:

    Personal _____

    _____

    Significant Others _____

    _____

    Professional _____

    _____

    Spiritual _____

    _____

    Humanitarian _____

    _____

    Other _____

    _____

3. Define your current responsibilities to:

Self _____

_____

_____

Significant Others _____

_____

_____

Community _____

_____

_____

Other _____

_____

_____

4. What role does your practice play in your ability to reach your goals?

Personal _____

_____

_____

Significant Others _____

_____

_____

Professional _____

_____

_____

Spiritual _____

_____

_____

Humanitarian _____

_____

_____

Other _____

_____

_____

5. What role does your practice play in inhibiting you from reaching your goals?

Personal _____

_____

_____

Significant Others _____

_____

_____

Professional _____

_____

Spiritual _____

_____

Humanitarian _____

_____

Other _____

_____

_____

6. How can you use your professional life to further your goals?
Personal _____

_____

Significant Others _____

_____

Professional _____

_____

Spiritual _____

_____

Humanitarian _____

_____

Other _____

_____

7. How can you overcome the areas in which your practice inhibits
you from accomplishing your goals?
Personal _____

_____

Significant Others _____

_____

Professional _____

_____

Spiritual _____

_____

_____

Humanitarian _____

_____

_____

Other _____

_____

_____

8. What personal qualities are required of the independent practitioner?

_____

_____

_____

9. Which of these qualities do you believe you have?

_____

_____

_____

10. How will these qualities assist you in developing your practice?

_____

_____

_____

11. If you believe you need to develop the qualities you have listed that you do not believe you have, how will you compensate?

_____

_____

_____

12. Comments:

_____

_____

_____

IDENTITY AND PRACTICE-BUILDING

In the end, in analyzing your own personality and needs, you will begin almost automatically to start thinking about business not as an adversary to whom you are hopelessly ill-suited, but as a natural extension of your personal identity, including the type of therapy you practice. Because relationship therapy is what we believe in, we see the business end of our practice as relationship-centered, too. Our business is based on caring, empathizing, and creating rapport. Going back to the old Rogerian tenet, connectedness can occur in the daily course of life. For example, you run into a neighbor at the nearby dry cleaning store. When you ask about his family, he mentions that his son in a neighboring city has been having problems. You tell him about a colleague in that city whom you know well and respect. You are not trying to give your neighbor a sales pitch or hustle business for your colleague (or yourself in the form of return referrals); you are attempting to assist a neighbor who has a problem. The connection is a human one between two neighbors, friends, and/or colleagues. For the most part, people are not going to decide to see therapists based on where they got their degrees or on what styles of therapy they practice. We sometimes get so sophisticated in our own field that we begin to look at certain aspects as marketable or not marketable, forgetting that when it comes to business, what is in vogue may be irrelevant; it is the relationship that counts.

This same principle underlies the business decisions you make with your colleagues. You care for your colleagues as people and not as production units. You deal with their feelings as well as behavior, taking into account their perceptions and values. Whatever business decisions you make, grow from the human connections you establish first.

BALANCE, NOT BURNOUT

The trick to creating, building, and maintaining an independent practice is to think *building* and act on these thoughts when opportunities present themselves, without going too far in the other direction and becoming a workaholic or a person who cannot refrain from being "on." The inability to balance all the important facets of your life, of which your practice is but one, will result in burnout. If your activities are rooted in your identity, however, and your dealings with people are rooted in the human connections you establish, there is less chance that you will burn yourself out. If what you are doing ceases to be fun, that is, satisfying, energizing, and motivating, and starts to be drudgery, you need to stand back and admit, "This isn't working for me. I've got to make some adjustments."

To discover the balance and to prevent burnout, Joan believes that every three to six months therapists should sit down with a few colleagues, with a supervisor, with their own therapist, or with a workshop group to assess how their personal and professional lives are going.

You get imploded all day long with all kinds of "stuff." You can work under white lights, go wash your hands between sessions, engage in all kinds of little distancing tricks, and other people's problems still rub off on you. You need to eat well, sleep well, exercise, and clean out your self regularly. Otherwise you wake up one morning, having helped all these other people, and you just choke.

PART II
Public Identity

2/
The "M-Word": Reconciling Therapist and Businessperson

It is time now. You cannot avoid it any longer. The fear greater than certification, more awesome than your first patient. . . . It is time to discuss marketing—the "M-WORD."

The therapist in us cringes: "Are we not too honorable, too transcendent, to delve into the mire of sales/marketing/advertising?" Following is a verbal portrait of the fantasy. Meet Harvey the Hard-Sell therapist. The scene is a cocktail party. Harvey is a guest. He corners the other guests one by one. Here is an excerpt of his encounter with Clyde.

Harvey (H): Hi! I'm Harvey Doe. I'm a therapist and I noticed that you keep looking at the bird sculpture on the coffee table. Little obsessed, eh? Fetish, perchance? You always use this obsession to avoid social encounters, don't you? Yes, I can tell that this is an old pattern with you. You use it quite frequently. I can tell.

Clyde (C): Uh, well, actually, no. Well, I mean, see, I'm an ornithologist and well. . . .

H: You know, we needn't be ashamed of our little foibles and idiosyncrasies. The experts, like me, say that we're all a bit crazy. And hey! That's why I'm here. You're lucky that we met. And wouldn't you know it? I'm having a sale on obsessions this week. Five sessions for the price of four. And a double-your-money-back guarantee if you don't have at least five minutes through the day when you are obsession-free. Is Friday or Monday better for you?

C: But Harvey, I uh, mean Dr. Harvey, I uh, really don't think that I, uh, well, have a problem.

H: Exactly. Boy! You are resisting. Proof that I am right. Not that I needed any. You are really worse off than I originally thought. Resistance and denial besides a serious obsession. Better not wait till Monday. I've got a spot on Friday used only by a little old lady for a mild case of nerves. We'll let you have her time. See you Friday at two.

   Here's my card. Oh, don't be late. I charge whether you're there or not.

C: Two on Friday. Well, uh thanks, I guess, Doc.

In the dichotomous thinking of helper versus entrepreneur, Harvey emerges as the bad-guy salesperson of our nightmares. He is also our revenge fantasy of how some successful-at-business therapists achieved their success. We console ourselves by thinking that these therapists have sold their souls to the devil in the name of profit and fame. In reality, there are few Harveys. Because we're afraid of becoming a Harvey, however, we sometimes "overcompensate" and do no marketing at all. Go to any of the professional meetings in your field and, although the situation is changing, you will still hear marketing talked about as a dirty word: the M-WORD. Beyond the fantasy, what does appropriate marketing of a professional practice entail?

We can't state this often enough: if you want to be in independent practice, you must start thinking of yourself as a businessperson as well as a therapist. You are selling a service—therapy—and to attract customers (patients) you must market your service. Other professionals—physicians, veterinarians, optometrists—have had to face a similar situation. As therapists, however, we have often faced self and societal expectations contradictory to the notion of selling this service called therapy. We have all had at least one client say to us, "You're only doing this because you get paid for it." Dutifully, we demur, until we have ourselves convinced that money means nothing to us.

If we stop, however, and are honest with ourselves, we have to admit that money is one way—certainly not the only way—we use to validate our therapeutic expertise, our education, and our training. For us to say to the mechanic who is repairing our car, "You're only doing this for the money," would be ludicrous. The mechanic would be highly unlikely to feel guilty; the "accusation" would be no accusation at all, merely a statement of part of the truth. Yes, the mechanic is doing the job for the money *and* because he or she is good at it, enjoys working with his or her hands, and feels a sense of satisfaction in the work.

We are no less entitled to payment for our services than is the dentist, the grocery store owner, or the person who delivers our newspaper, all of whom do their jobs for the money as well as for less tangible reasons. In fact, calling yourself a businessperson in independent practice is similar to being an employee of an agency: both involve a contractual relationship that provides a service in return for pay.

Traditionally, business has distinguished between services and products (or goods). Services are intangible, usually centered on actions rather than material objects. You cannot store services nor take inventory of them. Services are also more dependent on people, rather than on equipment or machinery. (These are broad distinctions. Think, for example, of the service implications of a restaurant's dishwashing equipment or an anesthesiologist's respirator breaking down.)

There are also differences in marketing a product and a service business. The distinction is not that the former must market its products while the latter simply waits for the customer to walk through the door; rather the difference lies in the marketing strategies that are most effective for a particular type of business. A general rule of thumb, for example, is that the more service-oriented the business is, the more marketing will depend on word-of-mouth advertising and personal referral rather than on media advertising to be effective. There are some types of businesses that require little marketing. These are usually in new, "hot" areas with little competition. As soon as enough people enter the field, or the area itself becomes more commonplace to the general public, the days of the seller's market are over.

In our own experience and those of many of our workshop participants, 20 years ago independent practice was the kind of service business in which you could hang out a shingle and wait for patients. The wait was not very long. Hanging onto this notion in the 1990s, however, ignores the reality that we are now in a buyer's market, and this kind of thinking will almost certainly result in failure of an independent practice.

We are not, however, advocating your turning into Harvey the Hard-Sell. Despite our stereotype of business being exclusively competitive, the history of American business is not just a tale of greedy robber barons driving others into bankruptcy and failure. Rather, American business also has a history of grass-roots networks of referral and mutual support. Many businesses began as small, family operations that grew because neighbors, shop owners, and the person who made deliveries used the service or product themselves and made referrals to others. Our marketing strategies are all based on a model of cooperation rather than competition. Of course, our cooperative model obliterates our competition! Cooperation is good business.

THE IMPLICATIONS OF COOPERATION

We firmly believe that in referrals "the more you give, the more you get." Too often, we worry about a limited supply of clients. In a way, such thinking undervalues our services and talents. To assume that few people will use our services is to judge these services as not very important. Even if there were not a huge population from which to draw, we would probably devise methods and techniques to meet a variety of needs: we would find a way to adjust to the market. (To reassure yourself that there is a substantial market, simply take a look at the size of the self-help/psychology section in your local bookstore. Although "in" topics may change, the public's overall interest in psychological issues has remained consistently high.) If all of us had completely full case loads, if every in-patient facility and out-patient clinic were operating at capacity, and if new therapists continued to stream out of graduate school at the current rate, there would still be under-served populations.

Both of us are quick to say to other therapists, "I want you to meet my friend, Ralph/Joan." Some of these people have responded by saying, "Why would I want to meet Joan/Ralph? She/he is in competition with me." We respond, "What do you mean, competition? There's more than enough to go around." We often receive calls from clients who say, for example, "Joan, I respect you, but I don't want to come and see you because you're this way or do that; I'm looking for this." We will send people to colleagues in our respective communities or nearby communities. (For example, some highly visible people in Tucson prefer to be seen by someone in Phoenix and vice versa.) There is enough to go around if we work together; if we are always competing, we look self-serving.

Joan once attended some meetings in Washington, D.C., concerning joint legislation and lobbying on the part of psychiatrists with representatives from CHAMPUS.* The main message from CHAMPUS was "quit competing with one another [in the mental health field]." One of the psychiatrists responded, "You shouldn't let those people [nonpsychiatrists] diagnose." The CHAMPUS representative replied, "I've seen some psychiatrists make some mistakes on diagnoses, too. Why can't you all work together?" This kind of competition is counterproductive for all of us—within the field, in the community, and to the public.

More important are the ethical implications of cooperation for our patients. It is inappropriate to assume that we can be equally effective for all patients. All of us have areas of particular competence—acknowledged or not—that best serve certain people. The same is true for our colleagues. Consequently, a professional network among practitioners who refer patients based on each others' strengths results in the highest quality care for the patient **and a better reputation for our field**—from which we all benefit. Joan asks, "How many of you know the

---

*Civilian Health and Medical Program of the Uniformed Services, a medical insurance program for military personnel and their dependents.

myth of Procrustes? Procrustes had a bed of a certain size. If you were too short, he stretched your legs; if you were too tall, he chopped them off! We have to guard against doing therapy this way. Most of us practice a particular type of therapy. When a potential client comes in, if we simply 'fit' him or her into our program, we are doing that person and ourselves no favor."

Frequently patients are surprised at Joan's intake procedure. She tells potential patients that the intake is an opportunity not only for the patient to assess whether Joan is right (appropriate) for him or her, but also for Joan to assess if the patient is right for her. Patients respond, "You mean even if I can pay you, you might not see me?" Joan says, "I mean even if you can pay me, I might not see you. If I think John Doe may be better for you, I will refer you to him." "But my doctor told me to see you." "Your doctor told you to see me because I do good intake work. We have two behavioral modification people who work with phobias. They will take you to a local hotel and work with you to overcome your fear of elevators. You may be in treatment for six months. If you work with me on an elevator phobia, it could take three years." Joan gets a reputation among her colleagues for not hoarding potential patients, and a reputation in the community for considering the patient's interests first. She also increases her success rate because she chooses those patients with whom she will work, and she chooses based on knowledge of her past success.

Ethically and practically, we think that developing appropriate, cooperative support is a necessity. Joan strongly urges therapists to have in place a system whereby they can reach a psychiatrist who will admit their client for evaluation within a few hours. She cites this example:

Late in the day, I got a call from a pediatrician who said, "Joan, I have an emergency. Can you see her?" I said yes and tried to find somebody in the office who could because I was booked. I couldn't find anyone, so at nine o'clock at night I let her into the office. She sat down and basically told me that I was going to put her into a trance, and she would be dead within the next 48 hours. She said these messages came to her in German and English. We spoke a little longer, and she began to hear a hymn and started to sing to me. I called Dr. R and said, "I need your help. I want to send you a lady." He said, "Okay, I'm here," and off the patient went. I don't have to worry about who walks in because I can call somebody within or outside my office and say I need help, need someone to back me up. Everyone in independent practice needs that kind of backup; you get that aid by knowing your colleagues professionally and socially. You build that kind of backup by deliberately seeking it out.

It is also important to establish a network among several disciplines. At various times, you may need to be in touch with physicians, attorneys, judges, or clergy. If a person came to see you in your role as therapist, but during the intake you noticed the person's arm was bleeding profusely, to continue to treat the person as though he or she had only a psychological complaint would be unethical. Therapists are not trained nor competent to give legal, medical, and financial advice; yet these areas may be entwined in a client's treatment. Joan states,

I find that two or three times a week I need legal information. I may know the answers, but common sense about liability issues tells me if I'm not a lawyer to keep my mouth shut. I have three or four lawyers in family relations, personal injury, divorce, and general law whom I can call and say, for example, "I've got a client sitting here who was poisoned by carbon monoxide from a furnace. Do you think it's worth his/her seeing a lawyer? Is this the kind of case for you or for whom would this case be right?" I never identify the lawyer to the client nor the client to the lawyer, so no one is in jeopardy. Some lawyers might automatically say, "My God! A free case!" but the ethical, competent ones who recognize the value of professional relationships will give you a realistic, truthful answer. When I call, I will say to them, "Hi, this is Joan and I'm working. May I ask you a question?" This is their cue that I'm not calling to have lunch or set up a tennis game.

This kind of access to other professionals is difficult, if not impossible, unless you have worked outside the office to cement your relationships with them.

Whether you are talking about cooperation between mental health practitioners or between practitioners and other professionals, the focus is on developing a team approach—as appropriate—to a particular client's problem. Ralph cites the example of dealing with a couple whom he is seeing in a family therapy context. The women cites her husband's alcoholism as a problem; the man denies he has a drinking problem. Ralph responds by saying, "I don't know if you're an alcoholic or not. Your wife says you are. You say you're not. It's a tie vote, and I'm not going to vote because I'm not a specialist. I would like you to see John Doe, a member of our group who does specialize in that area, for an evaluation. If he and you begin to agree that something needs to be done in that area, then I would like you to deal with him in that area." Ralph also co-leads groups with people who specialize in other areas. This kind of team approach helps to ensure that the patient gets the most competent treatment available. At the same time, the therapist expands his or her referral base by involving and staying in contact with other professionals.

DEFINING SUCCESS

If the first assumption underlying our marketing strategy formulation is the need to base it on your own personality, then the second assumption is the need to define success for yourself. Ideally your practice will be based not only on who you are but also on what you want. Endless techniques and instruments exist to assess your goals. You may find them valuable; however, what we are interested in right now is your personal, emotional definition of success. (In Chapter 3, we will look at success in a different way, giving you a "formula" for achieving marketing success no matter how you have defined the content of that success.)

The following questionnaire will help you clarify your definitions and priorities for personal and business success. You will use the answers to this questionnaire in formulating a marketing plan (see Chapter 4).

SUCCESS QUESTIONNAIRE

1. *Check any categories that apply and answer accompanying question(s).*

   Success for me includes:

   Community service _____ What kind? _____
   Control of schedule _____ Documented as _____
   Education _____ What kind and level? _____
   Freedom to take time off _____ How much per year? _____
   Money _____ How much per year? _____
   Number of patients _____ How many? _____
   Power _____ Documented as _____
   Prestige _____ Documented as _____
   Publications _____ What kind? How many? _____
   Referrals _____ How many per month? _____
   Requests from colleagues for consultation _____ What kind?
   How many? _____
   Time for family? _____ How much? _____
   Time for philanthropy? _____ How much? _____
   Requests for speaking engagements _____ From whom? How
   many? _____

   _____
   Other _____
   _____
   _____

2. The three most important items from above are:
   a) _____
   b) _____
   c) _____

3. The most important item from a, b, and c (Number 2 above) is:
   _____

4. To achieve Number 3, I would compromise:

   Community service _____ What kind? _____
   Control of schedule _____ Documented as _____
   Education _____ What kind and level? _____
   Freedom to take time off _____ How much per year? _____
   Money _____ How much per year? _____
   Number of patients _____ How many? _____
   Power _____ Documented as _____

Prestige _____ Documented as _____

Publications _____ What kind? How many? _____

Referrals _____ How many per month? _____

Requests from colleagues for consultation _____ What kind? How many? _____

Time for family? _____ How much? _____

Time for philanthropy? _____ How much? _____

Requests for speaking engagements _____ From whom? How many? _____
_____

Other _____
_____
_____

5. To achieve Number 3, I would not compromise:

Community service _____ What kind? _____

Control of schedule _____ Documented as _____

Education _____ What kind and level? _____

Freedom to take time off _____ How much per year? _____

Money _____ How much per year? _____

Number of patients _____ How many? _____

Power _____ Documented as _____

Prestige _____ Documented as _____

Publications _____ What kind? How many? _____

Referrals _____ How many per month? _____

Requests from colleagues for consultation _____ What kind? How many? _____

Time for family? _____ How much? _____

Time for philanthropy? _____ How much? _____

Requests for speaking engagements _____ From whom? How many? _____
_____

Other _____
_____
_____

6. The most successful person I know is _____

7. I define that person as successful because _____
_____

8. The person in Numbers 6 and 7 is successful in business? ___ personally? _____

9. Success for me is more important:

   in business? _____

   personally? _____

   cannot separate the two _____

   I am not really success-oriented _____

10. Others see me as successful. Yes _____ No _____

    because _____

    _____

11. I define success as _____

    _____

    _____

12. I am/will be successful when/because I _____

    _____

    _____

13. When I am successful, it will mean that _____

    _____

    _____

14. To achieve success, I must _____

    _____

    _____

    Why? _____

    _____

    How? _____

    _____

    When? _____

    _____

15. I inhibit my success by _____

    _____

    _____

It is important to define success concretely. Often, when workshop participants have been asked their definitions, we have had to help them focus. It is also important to recognize that your definitions will include both tangible and intangible facets.

Listening In

Ralph (R): What would you define as a successful indepen-
   dent practice?
Participant (P): A full case load.
Joan (J): What is a full case load?
P: Twenty-five.
J: Anything else?
P: Yes, personal satisfaction, professional satisfaction, recognition in the community, financial success. . . .
J: Do you know what "recognition in the community" means
   to you? Do you want to be Woman of the Year? We need to
   think about what it is, because if we don't figure out what
   "X" means, what it is we want, what success is to us, then
   we won't even know when we're there. It's similar to
   having a contract with a patient. The patient comes in and
   we work together so that the patient can decide what he or
   she wants to be different by the time he or she leaves. How
   is your practice going to be different? So, what is success
   in terms of recognition?
P: People consulting you for particular problems, giving you
   referrals, asking you to speak.
J: So, involvement in your community is recognition. Anyone else?
P: Making a significant difference in the families in the community and, at the same time, being able to pay your bills.
R: I'm glad you said being able to pay your bills.
J: But, you see, as counselors and social workers, particularly, you're not supposed to talk about the money part
   because it's not "nice." The money should simply come
   in automatically. Many people who go from agencies to
   independent practice forget to talk to prospective clients
   about the financial contracts they have, and then they
   worry about why they don't get paid. . . . Another definition of success.
P: Moving along a continuum to an eventual place of maybe
   40-grand a year without having to work more than 40
   hours a week.

J: Is that gross or net?

P: Well, it's somewhere between gross and net, because there's a lot of hidden elements that aren't really just going into business.

J: Such as? I mean, do you want to take home $40,000 or do you want to take in $40,000 and take home $9,000? There's a big difference.

P: I don't want my IRS return to reflect $40,000, but I want to be living at the level of $40,000, and I want to use every net I can that's legal that will allow me to do that.

J: You want to be able to make your money work like businesspeople do? Then you're not really looking to take home $40,000. So something for which your definition of success will have to allow is a good tax accountant. That's a specific provision that will help you get what you want.

R: Some other ideas about what a successful independent practice means to you?

P: Not worrying about that juggling act when people terminate and there's no one else.

J: Figuring out and handling the juggling act is important in several ways to defining success—doing your practice-building and having enough confidence to know there's going to be someone else; at other times, deciding how many patients to take—how many times have you taken too many? None of you? That's interesting.

R: Most of you are more secure than I am and I congratulate you—my own way of doing a practice is to "overbuild" it.

J: That's why Ralph and I have so many people in our practice.

R: I want to recommend that you think about it. I tend literally to "overbuild" always. Then I don't worry. If it's cut too close in an independent practice and something happens, your case load can drop rapidly. We have had some people in our group who just built their practices to exactly where they wanted them, and then if something went wrong—the stock market went down, a facility closed down, a referral source dried up—it caused extreme anxiety. We have set up our group to mitigate against sudden drop-off. We have eight people in our setup, each of whom has a specialty area unique to himself or herself. As a group, we also try to have the advantages of both independent practice and a clinic, as does Joan. We're not a clinic, yet we work very closely as a team. We do family therapy but have these individual specialties that can be separately marketed—chemical dependency/addictions, hypnosis, biofeedback, vocational exploration, sex therapy, forensic psychology, whatever it might be. I tend to keep more people referred to me than I could possibly see myself, and I tell people in my group—they do the same for me—that I'll always be referring to the rest of them unless all of a sudden my case load drops. I would become more selfish quickly if suddenly this flow of referral resources weren't there. If, when you start to define success for yourself in specific terms, you find that you don't want to worry too much about keeping a steady case load, then you will have to devise strategies to protect against sudden drop-offs.

As you can see from the previous discussion, you may have to work to define the concrete particulars of success. The more concrete you can get, however, the more likely it is that your definitions will suggest strategies to help you realize success. For example, your definition of success may include the opportunity to work with interesting families and make a positive difference in their lives. While this is an admirable aspiration, it does not give you any clues about how to realize it. If, however, after further reflection, you recognize that you are especially fascinated by working with families in which chemical dependency is a major issue, and have felt enormous satisfaction when you have worked successfully with this situation, then you have just identified a specific target market. And once you have a target market, specific ideas about how to reach that market will begin to occur to you. At this point, you may want to go back to your success questionnaire and check to be sure you have given the most concrete, specific answers that you possibly can.

WHAT DO YOU HAVE TO OFFER?

A third underlying assumption for development of successful marketing strategies is a precise understanding of the product or service. In psychotherapy practice, the service is a hybrid of the therapist's personality, character and experience; the theoretical or philosophical approach; and the techniques used that reflect this approach. What is unique about you and your approach? What are your particular areas of expertise? The answers to these questions provide the content for the marketing strategy. Who you are and what you do are what you are selling.

As you did with the Success Questionnaire, use your answers to the following questions to develop your marketing plan (see Chapter 4).

MARKETABILITY QUESTIONNAIRE

1. List three types of experiences that you have had that would be marketable (for example, worked with pregnant teenagers; have certificate in chemical dependency counseling; attended intensive continuing education seminar on child abuse):

   a) _____

   b) _____

   c) _____

2. List three skills you think are most marketable (for example, trained ability to read nonverbal communication; understanding of and ability to use systems theory in practice; ability to use Jungian sand tray):

   a) _____

   b) _____

   c) _____

3. List three services you provide that are unique (or at least uncommon) in the marketplace (for example, don't charge for intake and termination sessions; do psychometric testing for my own and others' clients; run a group for minority widows):

a) _____
_____

b) _____
_____

c) _____
_____

_____

The three questions in the Marketability Questionnaire are designed to help you distinguish yourself from other therapists in your locale by answering the question, "What do I have to offer potential clients that other therapists are not offering?" Once you define this clearly and concretely, as with the Success Questionnaire, you will have a clearer idea of your market and how you can reach these people. If you had trouble answering the questions, you may want to think about **what** you would like to be able to offer potential clients and **how** to go about offering it. You may need to go back to school or attend particular continuing education seminars. You may need to intern with a particular kind of practitioner or a particular facility. You may need to engage in activities different from your current ones. Do not fantasize only about what would be nice; develop a concrete strategy to realize it.

3/
"Plurking" Through the Network: Taking a Private Practice Public

"Plurking" is playing while working and working while playing. When we are working seriously there is still some enjoyment, a sense of playfulness, involved. At the same time, when we are playing, we still have some sense of our working selves. We both feel that learning how to plurk is key to a successful private practice. The beauty of this concept is that it prevents the almost schizoid feeling that we are two people: the worker and the "real" person or, as seen from a different angle, our old friends the entrepreneur and the helper. These two selves compete for time and attention, setting up a prime scenario for burnout. The plurker, on the other hand, is an integrated person capable of simultaneous productive concentration and enjoyment.

When presented with the concept of plurking, many people immediately think of the executive on the golf course, closing an important deal on the fifth tee. However, there is one requirement to defining this executive as a plurker: the person is plurking ONLY IF HE OR SHE ENJOYS PLAYING GOLF! That is the difference between what we do, what we hope you will do, and what Harvey the Hard Sell does. Harvey types will force themselves to endure any and every situation so that they can "work" it. That they are only doing something for the potential business is apparent to almost everyone; we absolutely doubt their sincerity and quickly lose respect for them. What we are saying is, on the one hand, be aware of opportunities to play (enjoy, be challenged, be engaged, etc.) when you are working, and, on the other hand, be aware that opportunities for work (contacts, referrals, information sources) can and will arise when you are playing.

For us, plurking is a way of life. We are not trying to say, however, that in order to be successful you must ascribe to plurking-as-life. For instance, we have been asked if we have any friends who are not referral sources. The answer is "of course." At the same time, though, we realize that referrals come from unexpected sources and circumstances, so we keep alert to the possibilities. Plurking is a skill that you can apply when and where you choose. You can establish a comfortable "plurk level" consistent with the values and goals you have already established. In thinking about how we can plurk in our lives, we find it most useful to ask, "What do I like to do that may also involve visibility for myself?" The idea is to become involved in activities or with people with which you would get involved anyway, whether or not you were trying to build a practice.

THE SUCCESS FORMULA

Visibility is a key focus in the working-while-playing mode of plurking. Previously, you defined for yourself the *what* of success; these goals, and the strategies to realize them, will be different for each person reading this book. One principle, however, underlies whatever goals and strategies you choose: $S = V_E \times T$—Success equals Visibility sub Exposure times Time. Visibility means that you are *seen*; exposure means that you *reveal* yourself in order to educate others about what you do and are. Notice we use the word educate rather than sell; marketing your business will be much less alien to you if you realize you are involved in the process of educating individuals and the community about therapy itself, and not just about you. Visibility/exposure is related to time as a ratio: the more time you have been in private practice (in a given geographic location within a given specialty area), the less work you have to do to be visible/exposed. Conversely, the less time you have been in private practice, or the less time you have been in a particular city or town, or that you have specialized in an area, the more you will have to engage in activities that give you visibility and exposure. Ralph has been in practice in Phoenix for 20 years. He no longer needs to spend five to eight hours each week meeting, for example, with different organizations or giving various talks.

Networking

The many ways by which we gain visibility and exposure usually involve networking. Without question, networking has been the "in" business concept of the era. Networking, a noun, has been twisted into a verb and parodied in the movies. Parody aside, networking is critical to marketing a professional practice. If we are uncomfortable with the idea of networking—everyone has some experience with its extremes after all—we may conjure up the image of Gladys the Gadabout (Harvey the Hard-Sell's cousin) who flits from meeting to meeting, passing out business cards, and rarely finds time to actually practice. In classically manic form, Gladys fills the room with reminders of her existence, but rarely, if ever, remembers your name. This is not the model we endorse. Networking is simply the process of making contacts through formal organizations and informal structures, which allows you to get referrals and clients and to provide these to colleagues. Through sharing information, you grow professionally and contribute to the growth of the therapeutic profession itself (see Figure 1).

The entrance point to the loop is the success formula. Visibility is the catalyst to the loop. What you do to make yourself known in the community is the process of networking. You interact with the community and it refers people to you. You refer clients to members of the community; you support their

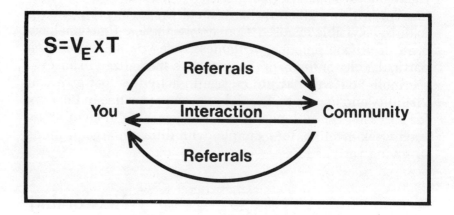

Figure 1. The Networking Loop

businesses and organizations. Notice that interaction is bi-directional. In other words, you cannot simply give a speech (interaction in one direction) and disappear. You need to be available for feedback (referral, consultation, follow-up activities) from the community (interaction in the opposite direction). Also, notice that the referral line on the chart is distinct from the interaction line. While you need to be active in the community to receive referrals, the referrals themselves result from your accumulated activity rather than any particular activity.

Of course, not every activity is equally useful from a networking standpoint. We have both discovered that by being involved in certain activities, not as therapists but as people who enjoy certain shared activities with particular groups, we keep running into the same groups of people. We emphasize that you meet people as people, as equals, in these situations; nevertheless, if you are networking with a large enough group of people regularly, you increase your chances that these people will think about you when someone they know needs a therapist.

Ralph enjoys jogging, but he has not built his practice around the activity even though he sometimes meets other people while jogging. This does not mean he must give up jogging because it does not build his practice; it does mean that he recognizes that his reasons for jogging have little to do with his practice, and he does not pretend he is building his practice when he is jogging. On the other hand, Ralph also plays golf. He belongs to two clubs whose membership includes the kinds of people his group practice tends to attract. We do not believe that people are going to be able to judge our therapeutic skills by meeting us on the boards of the symphony or the theater or in a sports league; they will, however, get a feel for us as people.

Ralph often quotes Virginia Satir who, when Ralph was in graduate school, responded in a letter to his inquiry, "What makes a family therapist? *The person qua person is more important than the methodology.*" This is the bottom line whether we are talking about what makes a good therapist or what makes an effective marketing strategy.

Positive and Negative Visibility

There are many different ways to be visible; anything that makes you visible contains some possibilities for networking though, as we have just pointed out, some activities are better than others. Do not overlook the *givens* of your life at a particular time. Some of Joan's best referral sources are people with whom she car-pooled when her oldest daughter was in nursery school. (Her daughters are now in their early-twenties.) These people know Joan not as a therapist but as a mother and a responsible car pooler; though these kinds of relationships are not overtly professional, they nevertheless have a large impact on the therapist's practice—an impact that can be positive or negative. Anytime you interact, you are perceived. We like to summarize this idea as "wherever you go, there you are." Whether you are in your Birkenstocks or running out in the rain in the middle of the night for a quart of milk with only your raincoat on and nothing underneath, there you are. Whether you want to be seen or not.

Frequently, in our workshops, when we talk about plurking, some therapists will say, "I don't want to do that, that's not me. I want to work from 8 to 4 or 5, then I want to go home, go hiking, sit with my family. I don't want to be aware always that I'm looking for clients." We are not trying to say that you should not have separate time for yourself. For most of us, some separate time is necessary. We are also not saying that you should run your whole life around what is best for business. We would become dangerously close to automatons or, worse yet, amoral Harvey the Hard-Sells, if all our decisions were only based on business. What we are trying to say, however, is that even if you do not want to be aware of potential clients, you must be aware that potential clients are looking at you. For example, when you go hiking and someone hikes by you, but you pretend not to see them because you are on your "off-time" and do not want to be invaded or bothered, what kind of message are you sending that person? What reaction does the person have to your message? What image of yourself are you leaving with that person?

Ralph tells the story of a therapist (not in his group practice but in an adjacent office) who had bug exterminators to his house one morning. Later that day, the exterminator was at the home of Ralph's group's office manager and said, "You won't believe it, but I was in the house of this psychiatrist this morning and he was carrying on and screaming and yelling and throwing things. Boy, was he crazy!" From the exterminator's description, the office manager recognized the psychiatrist to whom he was referring. How many other people did the exterminator tell?

Appropriate Behavior

Most of us who live in "small" communities have to be aware of how we package ourselves and where we are. The network is choked with grapevines. For example, Tucson and Phoenix are technically medium and large cities, respectively, but if you sneeze in the Tucson foothills on the northside in the morning, by afternoon people on the southside will know you have a cold; by the next day, they will know about it in Phoenix. Bad news travels faster than good news. If you are in independent practice, bad news about *you* can wipe you out quickly, and bad news about others in the field affects all of us. It is important that we keep our own noses clean and help each other do the same. We need to recognize what the average citizens of our communities—assuming for the moment that these people are our target market—regard as *acceptable* behavior. What is acceptable in Los Angeles may be frowned upon in Tucson and Phoenix. You may choose to step outside the acceptable context of a given community, but if you do, you need to understand and accept both the effects that this has on people's (read: potential clients') perception of the therapeutic community and the limits it imposes on your ability to market your own practice.

What we are really talking about here is the concept of *appropriateness*. There are many levels of appropriateness that apply to greater and lesser degrees. For example, the ethics codes of various professional organizations describe one form of appropriateness that applies across the board to all the members of the organization (and which nonmembers with similar kinds of training/practice will want to think seriously about emulating, even if they decide not to belong to the organization). Norms for appropriate dress, on the other hand, are usually specific to a given geographic area. For example, Ralph used to practice in Boston, where the dress tends to be more formal than in Scottsdale, Arizona. The dress that would tend to make people comfortable in Scottsdale would probably have the opposite effect in Boston and vice versa. Appropriate dress is also determined by such factors as the type of client your practice currently serves, the ambiance of your office, and your target market. You are probably going to experience a credibility problem if you show up at IBM in sandals; conversely, you may put off a group of teenaged dropouts if you show up for a presentation in extremely expensive or overly formal clothes. (Be aware, however, that you will probably experience the same problem if you try to dress like the teenagers themselves!) Again, we are not trying to make good and bad value judgments—at least about dress; ethics is another matter. What we are saying is to be aware always of the impact that going outside the norms of appropriateness will have on your practice, and plan your marketing strategies accordingly. If you feel very strongly, for example, about dressing a certain way, you may want to locate your practice (geographically or in terms of target market) where your way of dressing is appropriate.

TARGETING YOUR NETWORKING

To market your business successfully you need to target your market. One of the ways to do this is to target your networking. Networking is not just activity done for the sake of being in motion; it involves conscious decisions about the most efficient ways to get information you need, or to let key organizational decision makers know what you do, or to make individuals who have need of your specialization aware of your existence.

Some people confuse joining organizations—any organization will do, they think—with networking. If you join an organization and are not active, the result may be worse than if you had not joined at all. You may be perceived as noncommitted—a phony—and members may interpret your behavior as a rejection of them. That is one reason why it is important to be involved with people and groups with whom you share interests, because your involvement will be genuine.

There is another bonus to being involved with people around a common interest, which may sound a little silly: it gives you something to talk about. If you can talk about an interest you have in common with someone, you do not have to worry about talking about yourself. In our society especially, once people have a "normal" conversation going, talk of their work and professional interests almost invariably arises. You can integrate your networking goal seamlessly into this conversation with much greater effectiveness than if you started talking about yourself apropos of nothing.

At the same time, however, we do not mean to imply that you should limit yourself to individuals or groups with which you have something in common. For instance, you will probably have a lot in common with members of a professional association of therapists in your speciality area. Joining such an organization can be very important to your professional growth—one goal of networking. But the pool of referrals available from this group, a second networking goal, will probably be fairly limited because you all practice the same specialty. Therefore, another kind of group may better serve your second goal.

Increasingly, networking is occurring not only between individuals, but also between groups. An illustration of this is the cooperation that has developed between Joan's group and another group practice in Tucson. Not only do the two groups challenge each other to volleyball games and get together for other social occasions and professional development activities, they have also worked out cooperative agreements that have resulted in their obtaining a number of large contracts with EAPs and PPOs in town. As Joan says, "It's hard to compete with us because, between our two groups, we're 28 strong, we have English- and Spanish-speaking therapists, and we cover an enormous range of specialty areas. In addition, three of us triage for the two groups, thus increasing our overall availability."

You do not, however, have to be in a formal group practice to participate in networking between groups. One of our workshop participants described an informal association that she and a number of other solo practitioners in her town formed. This association networks with other formal groups.

In whatever arrangement you participate, it is our opinion that networking among groups is becoming almost essential for those who want to bid on contracts with small- and medium-sized corporations. Two groups getting together to co-bid contracts can create a much more attractive package for a company because the two groups can offer a range of services, specialties, and multiple locations. Additionally, co-bidding can make *capitation contracts* (that is, charging a set rate per employee, an arrangement that is fast replacing the fee-for-service contract) much more feasible. Because capitation contracts depend on obtaining a large number of clients to be profitable, two groups working together would be much more likely to be able to handle this client load. (Before you as a member of a group attempt to form such an arrangement between groups with a particular corporation, however, you may need to check the requirements of the corporation's insurance company. Usually, you can create a *joint venture agreement* between the two group practices to contract with the corporation. If the insurance company requires that a single employer contract with the corporation, a joint venture agreement will probably not work.)

REFER UNTO OTHERS— THE TWO-DIRECTIONAL FLOW

As our networking diagram indicates and as we have mentioned, networking needs a two-directional flow in order to work. Thus, networking is not exploitation; it is instead an exercise in mutuality. We provide referrals to colleagues and, in exchange, receive referrals from them. For us, the process comes down to this: **the more you give, the more you get.** The process starts as a dyad and ends as a myriad. An exchange between two colleagues can ripple out in numerous directions. Both of us have had the experience of answering the phone and hearing, "I got your name from X in Miami, who got it from Y in New York, who got it from Z who lives in Chicago and who heard you speak at a workshop in San Francisco five years ago."

It is important—from both ethical and business standpoints—to support those who support you. Even so-called competitors have more to gain from sharing information, services, and referrals than they have to lose. After all, how have various professional groups such as psychiatrists and psychologists attained legitimacy (read: status, financial remuneration, access)?—with group action that created a group identity in the public's eyes. If you are competitive, you are focused on your competition and not on yourself nor your business; that is, you are **reactive**, making decisions in light of what your competitor does, and not **proactive**, doing what is best for yourself and your business. You also need to use common sense. Make sure you believe in the other's product, whatever it is. If you do not use or refer to someone who is giving you referrals, the considerate thing to do, if confronted, is to let the person know why as politely as possible. Though obviously this is often difficult to ascertain up front, you should try to get a feel for a person's character, competency, ethics, and so on before you cultivate a referral relationship. Try to do your homework about another person's area of expertise, training, and experience. In other words, take the referral process seriously. Refer to whom you know and be known to those referring to you. Networking is not a substitute for professional competency.

The referral process can be intricate and take time to develop. Many professionals make the mistake of expecting instant rewards in the form of referrals for their networking efforts. If you speak before a Rotary Club or a church or temple and say, "Gee, it's been three weeks since I spoke and no one's come to see me," you are letting your feelings get "hooked into" in a way similar to what can happen in therapy itself. You can create a very oppressive situation for yourself that is unrealistic. You may not hear from anyone or five people may walk in the day after you do a presentation. Someone who heard you speak three years ago may suddenly call and make an appointment. There is no one-to-one correspondence between a single activity and number of referrals; rather you must focus on your overall activity and results. As William Nichols, former president of AAMFT, editor of *Family Therapy News*, and independent practitioner for many years, has put it (Personal Communication, October 1988), "You cast bread out on the waters without any expectation of immediate, total, or specifically predictable return." Nichols adds, "People are seldom just sitting around waiting for a therapist, so that when you speak, they'll find what they're looking for and come running to you.

If you get known and make an impression of trustworthiness and competence, they'll think of you **if and when** they need the kind of services you offer.''

Ralph once did a talk show in Phoenix on sexual addiction; the phones hardly stopped ringing. He was told that the response was highly unusual. That day, he just happened to hit on a topic on many people's minds—a matter of coincidental timing. Ralph also had a person walk into his office who had heard him speak 15 years before. The client needed help and found out Ralph was alive, functioning, and still in Phoenix, so she sought him out.

The quirkiness of the referral process underscores the need to establish positive name recognition. Yes, the more ways you can get your name in front of the public the better, but you had better make sure your name is associated with positive recognition. Otherwise you could find yourself being remembered 15 years later not for an impressive lecture but as the person who embarrassed the whole audience by making a joke offensive to the elderly.

Putting Your Referrals to Work: Record-keeping and Follow-up

To get the most from the referral process, 1) keep records and 2) follow up with your referral sources. Record-keeping is the raw data from which you can learn about the market you are attracting by monitoring who is sending you referrals, who your most active referral sources are, and what kind of person is being referred to you. To aid this process, we suggest you keep a list of referrals: name of the person, when the person called, who referred the person, to whom the person spoke, who the person saw the first time, and to whom the person was finally referred (if applicable). (See Appendix II for a sample referral form.) This list is useful for a variety of activities and analyses. For example, you can invite the people on the list to an open house, send them announcements of new groups you are forming, new specialty areas, new associates, and so on, use the people as contacts for various organizations of which they are members, and of course keep the list as a record for your follow-up responsibilities. You can also analyze who is sending you what kind of referrals and how often.

The Importance of Follow-up

Follow-up with referral sources is more than politeness; it is essential to the process, especially if you hope to obtain future referrals. The referring person is interested in the results of his or her actions. In addition, referral follow-up is an opportunity to thank the person for the referral and to keep your name in the referral source's mind. Sometimes, the client's treatment depends on a team approach and ongoing communication between, for example, the primary physician, an attorney, and the therapist. Too often, this team approach is overlooked.

In Ralph's group, with the client's and/or the family's written permission to waive confidentiality, the therapist communicates with the referral source and others who are going to continue to be involved in the family's life (for example, physicians, attorneys, judges, clergy). As a sex therapist, Ralph often sees people for a specific problem within some larger treatment context. Ralph will send a letter marked "Confidential" with a cover page stating, "Dear So-and-So. . . . Thank you for referring [client's name]. I have this person's written permission to communicate with you. If there is anything additional you would like me to know, please contact me and I'll do the same with you." Inside the cover letter, there is another smaller envelope stamped "Privileged Information, Only to be Opened by [referral source, physician, attorney, etc.]." In this envelope is a letter he has dictated (again, with the client's written consent) detailing how he sees the situation and stating his desire to work as a team with the person.

This strategy is important to developing that sense of connectedness discussed earlier and part of the ongoing process of working with referral sources. We have received feedback over the years from many of our referral sources explaining that they refer people to us because, in addition to being competent therapists, we let the referral sources know they are appreciated and we keep them apprised of the referral's status and situation.

How to Follow Up and Stay in Touch with Referral Sources

What kind of follow-up you do is an individual choice based on your personality. Some people invite their referral sources to lunch periodically or to open houses (discussed in greater detail pp. 64–66). As mentioned, Ralph often writes follow-up letters; Joan is more comfortable on the telephone, though she cautions that phone contact depends on the people involved. If you are calling someone who is not going to return your calls, then you are not covering yourself in terms of responsibility.

Joan has asked most of the people with whom she works to call her and say, "I'm referring so-and-so to you and wanted you to know." She notes the date in her calendar, and if she has not heard from the person within 10 days, she will call the referral source back to let the source know. If she has seen the person, she will let the source know this (with the client's permission) and thank him or her for the referral. If someone else in her group is seeing the person, she will let the referral source know this and, again, thank the source for the referral. She finds this strategy keeps her name fresh in the referral source's mind and usually results in additional referrals.

In addition, Joan and Ralph will suggest that their clients see a physician for a checkup. That is essential. She does not tell the client whom to see, but she will refer to her referral sources if so asked. This strategy affords additional legal protection. The therapist does not want to end up treating someone, for example, for a stress problem when in fact the client has a temporal lobe disorder (as was the case with a 14 year old she saw). At times, clients also ask for referrals to lawyers, accountants, mediators, and so on, which we provide. We then let these referrals know that we have recommended them.

Another way to stay in touch with referral sources is a termination follow-up letter. The therapist can write a letter to the referral source saying, "So-and-so is not coming in to see us anymore. Here are some of the things that happened (with client's/family's written permission, of course). I appreciate the referral, and if I can be part of a treatment team in the future, please don't hesitate to call, etc." If your referral source is a client, seek written permission of the new client to thank the original referring client. Some clients might not want the referring client to know they were seeing a therapist, so obtaining written permission protects you against a charge of violation of confidentiality.

Occasionally, you will discover—again, by analyzing regularly your referral list—that referrals from a particular source that were once abundant have begun to drop off. It is best simply to contact the person and try to find out why. Be straightforward, for example, saying something like "I noticed that two years ago you gave me "x" referrals, and last year it was "y," and this year it's even less. Is there something going on that I should be aware of?" In some cases, the decision has nothing to do with you: it could be that the facility at which the referral source works has contracted with a specific group for mental health services, or the source has changed directions or positions and has fewer occasions to refer. The problem could be miscommunication between a referral source and your support personnel. Joan had a situation where a source became annoyed because he thought a secretary was telling him that Joan was unavailable and had no openings for two days. In fact, the secretary planned to call another therapist, who would arrange for any referral to be seen within 24 hours. You need to make it clear to referral sources that you welcome feedback from them regularly, and you need to work to maintain clear communication among you, your referral sources, the support staff and your colleagues.

Giving Back to the Community

If you are an active networker with a large number of referrals coming in and going out, sooner or later you will have to deal with the issue of "nice person"—pro bono—work, specifically how much and what kind you want to do. Friends may ask you for free advice, which may cement your friendship but may also cause discomfort to both of you. You will be asked to do gratis work: seeing people with no insurance, giving assistance to social service agencies, giving presentations or seminars or writing articles for networking organizations to which you belong—the possibilities are endless. There are no rules governing your level of participation in these activities. You may choose to fulfill certain kinds of requests because you believe in their inherent value; in deciding about other requests, you will want to weigh the visibility and exposure you get against the time and effort required. You may want to keep in mind that the more serious you are about making sure that your clients who can afford to pay you actually *do* pay, the freer you are to engage in pro bono work for clients who cannot pay. (See Chapter 7, pp. 135–149, section on fees, billing, payment, and collections for a more complete discussion of this issue.)

Stylistic Subtleties

In addition to the basic, commonsense practices in networking that we have mentioned—acting ethically, being honest about what you can and cannot do, knowing those who refer to you and to whom you refer—are what we might call stylistic subtleties having to do with the psychology of networking. Ralph created the following role-play conversation with one of his workshop participants. Although it may seem an obvious example of what not to do, we have both had experiences with people who have done what Ralph is dramatizing. "Ralph" is discussing his need for referrals with a "doctor" with whom "Ralph" has worked a couple of times in the past and is trying to persuade to refer to him:

Ralph (R): Say, Bill how are you doing?
Participant (P): Quite well, thank you.
R: I want to share something. You know that I do marital and family therapy and I'm really hurting right now, just don't

seem to have any patients. Since we've worked together in the past, I'd like you to know my situation and can you help me out?

P: How far are you from our emergency room? Well, I'd be glad to keep you in mind. Why don't you give your name, address, and phone number to my secretary?

R: Okay. You know I've been going through a lot of problems in my marriage, my wife has kicked me out and the divorce will cost me a lot of money. I've stayed pretty busy but I need to get busier right now. I know you're a caring person and I really need referrals right now.

P: Do you need some time to talk?

R: Well Bill, I'd like to talk, but right now I'm so busy trying to build my practice and stay ahead of all my financial needs, but please remember I do need to have more clients, okay?

P: I'll do that.

After this dialogue, the participant pointed out to Ralph and the rest of the workshop participants that he probably would not have sent clients to "Ralph" based on this interaction alone. Rather, whether or not he referred would be based on the nature of his ongoing relationship with "Ralph." The prospects for "Ralph" would be uncertain at best.

Actually, we could never see ourselves speaking this way. Not because "Ralph" was not telling the truth, but because it is the opposite of the attitude and behavior it takes to build a practice. Coming from such an overt position of need as "Ralph" does in this dialogue is probably going to make people very uncomfortable and immediately ready to question your professional ability, at least at this point in your life. It is similar to telling a new client at an initial session that you are really glad to see him/her because you need him/her or financially you are hurting or you have gone through something like he/she is going through.

It is important in the networking process to maintain a positive image of yourself as a successful person in demand. We are not trying to say you should lie or fake your way through a contact saying, "Oh, I've got a successful practice, and I can't see you for several weeks," when in fact you have nothing on the calendar. But neither is it useful, for example, to say to a client setting up his/her first appointment, "When would you like to come in? I can see you anytime this week, any time of day, 8, 9, 10, 11. . . ." Too often the person will respond with "I'll call you back later." Instead, say, "Would you like to see me Tuesday at 10 or Wednesday at 3?" This way you are responsive to the client's needs without sending "rescue me" messages. To be successful in independent practice, it is important to have a sense of realistic power, being in charge, and confidence that you will succeed. With clients, and occasionally referral sources, you do not want to appear more nervous than they are or you risk making them more anxious than they already are.

Workshop participants created the following role-play to illustrate a more effective way of asking for referrals. Notice that it communicates a request without the neediness of "Ralph." "Sue," a therapist, heard "Jane," an OB/GYN, speak at a public seminar. Sue arranged a follow-up meeting with Jane.

Sue (S): Dr. Smith, thank you for meeting with me. I enjoyed your presentation last week. I understand much of your practice deals with PMS. I wanted to let you know that I have been running a weekly group for the last two years for women who suffer from PMS. I think we have an excellent opportunity for cross-referral.

Jane (J): That's great to hear. I often feel I don't have enough time to deal with the psychological aspects of the problem with my patients. Tell me a little about your training and approach.

(Jane and Sue discuss their work.)

S: I would love to give a talk to your patients. If this makes sense to you, how could we set it up?

J: It does make sense. Let's set up a time with my secretary and work out the details. I would also like to sit in on one of your group sessions to get an idea of who would best benefit from them. I have a few patients whom I might be interested in sending to you.

S: You're welcome to come next Tuesday at 7. After that, we can determine which of your patients might be most appropriate for the group. I'll call your secretary tomorrow morning to set up an appointment. Thank you. I think we'll work well together.

J: I agree. I'm glad to have met you.

This approach works for several reasons. First, Sue has done her homework. She has not selected just any OB/GYN, but one whose work fits her specialty. She has heard Jane speak and has researched her practice to find where their work intersects. She communicates first **how she can help Jane,** not how Jane can help her. She immediately suggests an action with little risk to Jane. She gives Jane the opportunity to see her work before Jane commits specific patients for referral. This approach is both considerate of Jane and indicative of Sue's confidence and competence. She reinforces her interest by establishing specific dates and follow-up.

In the 1990s, therapists will have to be increasingly creative in devising ways to interact with people who can provide referrals. Many workshop participants have pointed out to us that cold-calling does not work anymore. Especially solo practitioners who work in large cities sometimes find that even when they work hard to keep themselves visible through follow-up letters and phone calls, they are forgotten two or three months later in the large pool of therapists. One therapist cited a situation in a large southeastern city in which EAP directors had stopped attending ALMACA (Association of Labor-Management Administrators and Consultants on Alcoholism) meetings because, in her words, "the providers have hit on them so much. You have to find more obscure ways to get to know people and let them know you as a person." This particular therapist offers herself as a speaker to personnel conventions and addictions conventions. She says that often people will come up to ask her questions and then she can find out who they are. They are already familiar with her specialty because she has spoken about it. She does get referrals in this way, but "there's no magic . . . it's hard work."

GETTING THE WORD OUT—
ADDITIONAL WAYS TO NETWORK

We have pointed out general principles of networking and mentioned a few suggestions for networking; we would now like to offer additional ideas for ways to network.

Advertising

The issue of advertising and its effectiveness frequently comes up in our workshops. We have mixed feelings about and have had mixed results from formal advertising. In a number of workshops, when asked to cite strategies that did not work as marketing tools, many people mentioned direct mail, one form of print advertising. It has been a general maxim in marketing that the more intangible your product, the more personal contact and personal recognition is required to sell the product; conversely, a tangible, concrete product will benefit most from advertising. Although as a general guideline this principle is probably true, specific situations can contradict it.

Certainly, we find the professional announcement useful in terms of creating name recognition. If we bring someone new into our group, we send an announcement with the person's name and specialty. The announcement creates name recognition for the new person and, for those of us in the group already known in the community, the announcement is a reminder of our presence. Obviously, moving your practice would be another situation in which you would want to send an announcement, also reminding people about your specialty area(s). Another kind of announcement we find useful is the specialty list, which names each of the people in the group and their particular specialty. And you could add a brief explanation of each area.

The notion of specialty announcements relates to another form of advertising—Yellow Page listings. We both list under several different relevant categories. Ralph has found that the most specific of his listings, Sex Therapists, has brought the most referrals, perhaps because of all the categories under which he lists, in metropolitan Phoenix that category has the fewest number of practitioners. Joan also believes it is important to list under a professional association, such as American Association of Marriage and Family Therapists, if one is included and you are a member. Such a listing implies a level of expertise and credentials not apparent in more general listings.

You might say, "In a whole year, I only got three or four clients from that listing." Those few clients will pay the cost of the ad, and it is quite likely they may do more than that in terms of networking and referrals. William Nichols (Personal Communication, October 1988) points out that, although he has gotten very few clients as a direct result of being listed in the Yellow Pages, a Yellow Page ad is important to credibility. He believes it is important that potential clients be able to find you in the Yellow Pages after they have obtained your name elsewhere and are considering seeing you. As an example, he cited his move from Florida to Michigan. The timing of the move was such that it was 18 months before his Yellow Page listings came out. He said, "The statement, 'I couldn't find you in the Yellow Pages,' came up fairly frequently from new clients who had been given my name. I'll always use Yellow Page ads if I'm in practice, not to get referrals or business but to be visible and, hence, reassuringly legitimate to those who already have my name."

Radio, TV, Newspaper Columns, and Books

The *specialty* principle may also hold true for radio and TV appearances or newspaper articles. Ralph has found it useful to get to know the programming director of radio and TV stations. (Do not forget the possibilities of public-access and educational cable TV.) Ralph then sends his group's specialty list to the programming director. When something happens in the community, which is what the director keys into, he or she starts looking around for somebody who can talk about, for example, child custody, or mediation, or domestic violence. Ralph has made himself useful enough in the past to programming directors so that now he has several directors who will automatically call and say, "Ralph, I need a person who can talk about this." If Ralph knows someone with expertise in the area, and can help the director do his/her job, he will eventually see the result in his practice. For example, Ralph made an appearance on the Phil Donahue Show. In that one appearance, Ralph reached a vast audience of millions—certainly a practice-building approach!

Writing an article or a column for a newspaper, a local magazine, or a newsletter is another effective networking technique. Obviously, the more regularly you can write for a publication, the more name recognition and credibility you develop with the reader. While writing an article here and there or writing a letter to the editor in and of itself may not be enough to bring someone in, these more sporadic activities can trigger name recognition if the person has heard of you or known of you in other contexts.

Since the publication of his book *Lonely All the Time* about sexual addictions, Ralph has experienced more name recognition and referrals. Obviously, a book with widespread distribution will provide opportunities for networking on a national level. Ralph also points out that while the *product*, the book, helps his networking efforts, the *process* of writing provides a creative outlet not tapped in his therapy practice and helps him avoid burnout.

Robert Schwebel, a therapist in independent practice in Tucson, illustrates how one small writing activity can lead to larger and larger ones (Personal Communication, December 1989). A number of years ago, Schwebel wrote a monthly article for a small co-op newspaper. At the time, he was taking a Spanish class and became friends with a person who happened to work at one of the two daily newspapers in Tucson. The friend showed Schwebel articles to an editor, who was enthusiastic about the idea of Schwebel writing a weekly column but rejected it because of lack of space. A number of months went by, and suddenly the newspaper contacted Schwebel and asked him to begin writing a weekly column.

Over the seven years that Schwebel has written the column, it has evolved to being focused mainly on relationship issues. Schwebel pursued writing for the newspaper primarily because he wanted to carve a writing niche for himself, not necessarily because he wanted to build his practice. As director of a local agency for three years and as an active public speaker, Schwebel already had a strong referral base. Nevertheless, the column has brought him substantial name recognition and referrals.

One day a producer from a small TV station in Tucson contacted Schwebel to request his help in figuring out topics for a public affairs show. He began as a consultant to the show. The producer was so impressed with his work that she asked him to be in the audience so his contribution could be recognized. Then she asked him to appear as a guest; finally she helped him make a demo tape as host of a show. Soon after, she left town, and Schwebel put aside his tape. Some months later he received a call from a hospital asking him to give a talk about relationships. Time constraints prevented him from giving the talk, but he did reference his newspaper work and the demo tape. Soon, the hospital had agreed to sponsor a TV show. Even with a sponsor, it still took months to get the half-hour, weekly show on the air. Although the show was very popular, after eight months of an increasingly grueling production schedule, Schwebel stopped doing the show in order to concentrate on two books he was writing.

Interestingly enough, Schwebel is not sure how much effect the TV show had on his practice, if any, in part because he was not looking for new clients at that time (Personal Communication, December 1989). Although he thinks the newspaper column had a much greater effect than the TV show, he attributes this discrepancy in part to the difference in time spent doing the activities—seven years of the column versus eight months of the TV show.

Schwebel points out that the newspaper and TV experiences have both provided extremely useful training for the promotional activities he must now do for his books, *A Guide to a Happier Family* (about relationships) and *Saying No Is Not Enough* (about raising children in an age of drugs). When these are finished, Schwebel sees himself moving back into some kind of TV work and writing more books, thus creating a kind of cyclic flow to his actions and, as with Ralph, providing him with a balance to his therapy sessions with patients.

Community Visibility

We have mentioned community service and education activities: serving on boards, doing other kinds of volunteer work, giving lectures, workshops, demonstrations, and seminars. These activities can be directly related to your work (lectures on your specialty, donated therapy sessions, etc.) or they can run far afield. You may think that general volunteer work is less valuable to practice-building than is an activity directly about your work, but this is not the case. As you give others assistance through the theater, the symphony, the crisis shelter, or Little League, people see you are available, they see you in public, walking and talking, they see you do not have horns, and they say, "Ah, I can refer to that person" or "That person may know where I can get some help." In other words, you convey the impression of **trustworthiness as a person,** and this impression includes the professional aspect of your life.

Related to this idea of general community visibility is the notion of keeping up with what is going on in your community (as well as with state and/or national trends). Too often, we get caught up in what is going on within our profession or specialty and forget about the larger world. For instance, Tucson and Phoenix, as high-tech Sunbelt cities, experience a lot of migration, both in and out of the state. Relocation is a big issue in both communities, an issue which also presents opportunities for therapists. Because of her husband's work at the University of Arizona, Joan was often asked to show spouses of people being recruited by the University around the community. After people committed to the University, Joan would often help them find houses, meet people, get on community boards and involved in other community activities. "It was my pleasure to help these deans, vice-presidents, and department heads because they're going to come in and run whole colleges and departments. One new dean accounted for something like 42 referrals in the following year. I get to help Tucson and myself at the same time."

One therapist we know was asked to take a leave of absence from his regular practice to work exclusively on relocation issues with employees of a large company that was shutting down certain operations in the Southwest. Similar to changes in the community, state or national changes in family demographics, in employment levels and types, in the stock market and the dollar, and in real estate can have implications for the therapist's practice.

Of course you could also look for volunteer activities that relate directly to your work. One of our workshop participants mentioned that she was referring large numbers of domestic cases involving child custody battles because psychologists were having to make do with pro bono evaluations. She wanted to find people who were interested in doing these evaluations. Joan suggested to another therapist who was looking to build her practice that she send a cover letter and résumé to the workshop participant and then follow up with a phone call expressing her interest in doing these evaluations. Why should the therapist do this pro bono work? Because when the therapist gives, her work is noticed and the referral source is happy with it and the therapist gets court experience, then the referral source also socializes and talks to a lot of lawyers and says, "I had [this therapist] do this work for me and it was great." Suddenly, this therapist's name is before a large number of lawyers who refer and that is the way you build a practice. (This process assumes, of course, a satisfied customer.)

Many civic and charitable organizations are constantly looking for speakers to address their regular meetings. Look for organizations whose charitable interests relate in some way to your area of expertise. For example, if you have expertise in addictions counseling, you might speak before a Lions Club meeting which currently focuses on drug awareness programs.

Cross-marketing

Networking may lead you to possibilities for *cross-marketing* with either another therapist or a related professional whose practice somehow dovetails with yours. Cross-marketing is the practice of combining resources with another person or institution for marketing, with the goal of generating more business as a result of the association. For example, think of "Sue" and "Jane" whose networking dialogue appeared earlier in this chapter; both dealt with the problems of PMS, Sue from a psychological perspective and Jane from a physiological perspective. Marketing themselves together could give each of them an edge with their respective markets because they would each be offering something more than their medical or therapeutic counterparts do.

Open Houses

Another networking technique we have found effective is the open house or breakfast. Again, though, if you expect a lot of people to begin automatically coming to your office or referring to you just because you have an open house, you are probably going to be disappointed; it just does not work that way.

The open house should reflect your image. In other words, do not expect to get many referrals if your fee schedule says "high class," but your open house—your promotion, the food you serve, the decor, the atmosphere—says "shabby" or "cheap." Clashing images can produce backlash instead of growth. Bottles of pop and chips and dip from the grocery store, unless you are at the lower end of the overhead/fee spectrum will not do. When we have open houses, we make sure we are conveying an image consistent with our practice as a whole: We have the event catered; we send printed invitations; our dress and the office's decor are neat, clean, and appropriate.

Ralph will sometimes "piggyback" two networking events: his group will hold an open house from 4 to 7 in the evening for which the mailing is huge—in order to foster name recognition, even among those who do not attend the event itself. Sometimes 350 people will attend. After the open house, a select group of about 40 people from the open house has been invited to go out to dinner at a good restaurant. These people are often those who have been particularly good sources of referrals in the past or who may be expected to be good sources in the future. Some people have been skeptical of the effectiveness of this two-part event, citing the expense of both an open house and dinner; but, as with other networking techniques, if you receive four or five referrals who subsequently become patients, you will have paid for your open house/dinner and gotten an enormous amount of "free" visibility.

When you have an open house you do not just invite neighbors, you invite people who have been good to you professionally—also former and current clients—to thank them. (Use your referral lists!) Also, target people you want to know—invite attorneys or physicians located near you. Not only will you create opportunities for yourself, you will also help these people make contact with each other. In their subsequent dealings with each other, your name may come up yet again. Even if they do not attend, you will have begun to create name recognition. Calling the people you have invited a week or two in advance to tell them you are looking forward to seeing them can also help boost attendance. A few cautionary words—be cognizant of your scheduling. One of our workshop participants told of her group's first open house—she can laugh about it now—which they inadvertently scheduled on Yom Kippur. ("We got a thank you note from the League of Arab Psychiatrists.") The group still occasionally gets fallout from that blunder. You might also think about scheduling an open house or party or breakfast during an unusual season. Everyone has Christmas parties. People get sick of them, and you probably will not get as much mileage from them as you would if you had a Valentine's Day party or Halloween party. One medical group in Ralph's area gives a Halloween party every year at which the staff dresses in costume.

Another potential trap—though this is a bigger problem for

small gatherings than for large—is hostility between two of your guests. William Nichols described [Personal Communication, October 1988] a classic blunder by an acquaintance of his who, as a new sports information director, invited the sports editors of the two local dailies to lunch. It was only when seated that he learned the two editors did not speak to one another. An awkward time was had by all. Before you plan an activity, try to find out if the people involved get along with each other.

DEVELOPING YOUR PERSONAL PLURKING STYLE

Plurking is really at the heart of the idea of independent practice as a lifestyle rather than as a job, a career, or even a vocation. We hope that after reading this chapter you can see that the plurking style you develop should be as personal as your therapeutic style.

Joan often uses a travel metaphor to describe her unique plurking style. She says,

There are many ways to get from one place to another. Some people ride a two-wheeled scooter—metaphorically speaking, of course! Some people drive a Ford or Chevy; still others prefer a Cadillac or Rolls Royce. I ride in a helicopter. Though there are some people who think it's a space ship, it is really just a helicopter. But that helicopter allows me to rise above the traffic—above the scooters, Fords, or Caddies—and see things others do not see. I always have the option of choosing one of the more usual vehicles if I need or want to, but the helicopter is my ticket to the big picture.

4/
Mapping Your Success: Marketing Plans and Specialties

Professionals are in the advantageous position of being able to market themselves as experts and consultants and less like individuals with something to sell. In the preceding chapter, we hope that we convinced you that "marketing-is-survival" for the business. In this chapter, we address the components of a marketing plan and examine how they work. In addition, we discuss the marketing aspects of specialization—the why and the how-to—using examples from a variety of specialties: sports psychology, spirituality, and childhood trauma therapy. We also discuss the relation of developing a specialty to career stage.

THE MARKETING PLAN

Marketing is a three-tiered process of **analysis, goal setting, and implementation.** In previous chapters, we looked at personal traits and an individual's uniqueness in the marketplace. You can integrate this data with basic marketing principles to develop a marketing strategy specifically designed for you. Your personality determines the style of your marketing strategies while your marketable qualities and the service of therapy supply the content of the marketing plan. The information that you generated about your definitions of success determines the limits of your business and, in turn, the type and amount of marketing you need to do. All of this information underpins the marketing plan.

Technically, the marketing plan is a document derived from the process of planning your marketing strategy. While the document serves as a guideline, it is the planning that is essential. For this reason, you might choose to contract a marketing research consultant to draw up the plan, but you will be remiss if you are not actively involved in the planning process. The plan itself is composed of three sections:

1. Situational Analysis (therapist's needs/market needs)
2. Marketing Objectives (goal setting)
3. Marketing Strategy (implementation) (Warmke, Palmer, and Nolan, 1976)

1. Situational Analysis

This section relates to earlier discussions of your personal and professional goals in relation to the market. That is, what do you want and how do the number of potential clients, the competition, and your access to the potential clients match up? The situational analysis includes statements about:

1. Your goals:
   a. The answers to your needs assessment in Chapter 1.
   b. The answers to the success questionnaire in Chapter 2.
2. Analysis of your services (refer to the marketability questionnaire in Chapter 2):
   a. What are your credentials and experience?
   b. Do you have a particular area of expertise?
   c. Are you in solo or group practice?
   d. What is your therapeutic conceptual base (Adlerian, Rogerian, transpersonal, eclectic, etc.)?
   e. What are your professional affiliations?
3. Target clients:
   a. Who are your potential clients? (families, women, corporate executives, etc. Be as specific as possible.)
   b. Group, individual therapy or both.
   c. How many clients constitute a full caseload?

4. Demographics of your area:
   a. How many potential clients of your targeted group live in the area where you practice?
5. Competition, direct and indirect:
   a. How many therapists with the same or similar credentials are practicing in your geographical area?
   b. How many therapists of any type are practicing in your geographical area?
   c. How many competing clinics/hospitals are there in your area?
6. Market attitudes in your community:
   a. What is the public attitude in your locale toward therapy and therapists?
   b. What is the general reputation of therapists?
   c. What is the public attitude toward your specialty?
   d. How generally known are you in your community?

CASE EXAMPLE: KALA

The following is a situational analysis for a fictitious therapist. We will also examine her marketing objectives and marketing strategies following each of the next two sections.

Kala is a chemical dependency counselor from a southwestern city of 500,000. She has been in practice for 12 years, the last three exclusively in chemical dependency counseling. She has undertaken a marketing plan to focus her goal of expanding her practice.

Analysis of Services

Kala holds an M.A. in counseling psychology and a certificate in chemical dependency counseling. Her expertise includes codependency and cocaine addiction in women. Throughout her career, she has been a solo practitioner. Her office is located in a professional office complex within two blocks of a medical center. Her clinical approach is eclectic but based on 12-step programs. She is a member of ALMACA, the Chamber of Commerce, and Business and Professional Women (BPW).

Target Clients

Kala believes she works best with women and teens who have problems with cocaine addiction and/or codependency. She would like to limit her practice to these areas. She concentrates on group therapy but offers individual sessions to group members who need them. Kala requires individual intake and termination sessions with all of her clients. Her current case load consists of three groups of 10 members per week. Clients may attend more than one group per week.

Demographics

According to local health department statistics and the calculations of a local chemical dependency treatment center, there are 20,000 potential clients in Kala's city.

Competition

Kala's direct competition includes 12 individual chemical dependency counselors and five inpatient treatment centers listed in the phone book. Her indirect competition includes an additional 34 therapists who do not specialize in dependency, but who may be called upon by their clients to treat it. (These therapists could serve as referral sources.) There are three general mental health facilities in the area.

Market Attitudes

The public attitude toward chemical dependency therapy is generally supportive, as is that of the medical community, evidenced by the large number of treatment facilities in the area. Local mental health organizations offer monthly educational programs focused on different aspects of chemical dependency, and these are almost always attended to capacity. In her workshops, Kala is often asked about special programs for women; after doing research, Kala has also found little public information that is targeted to women. Most of Kala's clients come from physicians' referrals. She is somewhat visible in the larger community.

2. Marketing Objectives

These objectives are time-based, observable intentions. They reflect the situational analysis in that they refer to your goals and present your attainable ambitions, given the market demographics, attitudes, competition, and accessibility. Effective marketing objectives are stated precisely and with measurable outcomes. Typically, marketing objectives consider the following:

1. Size of the practice:
   a. What is the maximum case load desired?
   b. What is the target date for achievement of goal? (e.g., "The practice will serve 25 clients by September 25.")
2. Specific indication of services—current and projected:
   a. Exactly what services do you now offer?
   b. Are there new services you wish to offer?
   c. What is the target date of new services? (e.g., "In addition to the current caseload of 10 individuals per week, I will see five families and conduct two groups by May 4.")

KALA'S MARKETING OBJECTIVES

Kala wants to increase the size of her practice and focus on women and teens as the target population for her services. Thus, Kala's goal (marketing objective) is to conduct five groups of 12 clients per week. Members will be charged $40.00 per group session. She plans to achieve her goal in nine months.

3. Marketing Strategies

Given your situation, that is, the work you do in your particular community, strategies are the specific formulations you devise to meet your objectives. Many therapists consider this part of the marketing process to be the most creative and enjoyable. The specifics of networking and referral generation discussed in Chapter 3 provide ideas for developing your marketing strategy. Look for activities that let colleagues and the public know that you exist as a competent and caring practitioner. In considering the strategies, the wise marketer analyzes his or her current and past practices, looking for what has worked in the past and what has not. Before you develop the third part of your marketing plan, you may want to consider the strategies that have been successful (meaning they generated either clients or contacts who subsequently referred clients to you), and those that did not seem to work very well. The "Follow-up" category is included to nudge you to speculate on a way to rework or retry the strategy for more success. Keep these in mind when you work on your new marketing strategies.

	Past Strategy	Outcome	Follow-up
1.			
2.			
3.			
4.			
5.			

Preparing marketing strategies requires you to answer the questions posed in the situational analysis and marketing objectives and to create the means to those ends. An efficient way to conceptualize strategies is to list the objectives you developed and then brainstorm some possible techniques to realize each objective.

KALA'S MARKETING STRATEGIES

In order to meet her goal of expanding her practice, Kala must become more recognized in the community and garner more referrals from her colleagues. Kala admits she knows little about marketing and developed the following strategic plan from what she called "simple logic and a little risk-taking."

Notice how her plan is comprised of simple, measurable steps with specific times for completion.

1. List all mental health treatment facilities that specialize in drug and alcohol treatment, by Friday.
2. List all local treatment facilities that are not specifically set up for drug and alcohol treatment but might encounter patients who need that help, by Friday.
3. List everyone I know who is associated with the facilities in #1 and #2. Arrange to discuss their needs and the link to my services with at least five of them in the next month.
4. Arrange within two months to present a talk at the Chamber of Commerce and BPW [organizations to which she belongs] on the special needs of women who are addicted and/or how to recognize problems in teen-agers.
5. Offer to do a program with the local news-talk radio show about how to identify addictions in self and teenage children. Contact programming director by next week. Do this within one month of the radio interview.
6. Write a guest column for a daily, weekly, or monthly local newspaper on one issue that comes up during the talk-show interview. Do this within one month of the interview.
7. Offer to speak at the Parents' Club of my daughter's school before the end of this semester.
8. Document change in practice after each step, and at three-month intervals.

Discussion

If you look back at Kala's complete marketing plan, you can see how each section proceeds logically from the previous section. The marketing plan, then, is the record of your data collection about your goals, the feasibility of meeting those goals in the market in which you are located, and the means by which to achieve those goals. In preparing a marketing plan, however, you do not have to rely exclusively on your own creativity if you do not want to. There are a number of ways to learn about research marketing techniques for small businesses and professional corporations. In addition to consulting marketing books or hiring a marketing research specialist in your community, you might discuss techniques used by your successful colleagues or plan a marketing forum with local experts for one of your professional association meetings. Most communities of at least moderate size offer "entrepreneurial training" programs for the small businessperson. Economic development corporations, which are often branches of local government, are becoming more interested in helping small businesspeople. The federal Small Business Administration (SBA) also conducts seminars in marketing and offers excellent materials on marketing topics. Under the auspices of the SBA, the Service Corps of Retired Executives (SCORE) offers free, individual consulting to small businesspeople. (See also Suggested Readings on p. 197 for marketing resources.)

FITTING THE MARKETING PLAN TOGETHER

CASE EXAMPLE: MAX

Now that we have gone through the three components of a marketing plan, we would like to show you how they all fit together. We created the following marketing plan for another fictitious therapist, Max. Max is an art therapist from a rural northeastern town of 35,000. Psychological services are limited to a crisis wing of the community hospital and three independent practitioners: a psychiatrist, a clinical psychologist, and Max. He has been in practice for eight years. His goal in developing a marketing plan is to expand his practice into the smaller, more rural communities within a 100-mile radius of his town.

1. Situational Analysis

Analysis of Services

Max is a registered art therapist with a specialization in child development. After three years with a group practice in a metropolitan area, he returned to his home town and established a solo practice. He tends to work with individuals but will conduct family sessions with the local psychologist, a family therapist, if the need arises.

Target Clients

Max decided to specialize in the treatment of children both because he feels that he works very effectively with them and because the community provides few services for them. The more rural areas, which he is targeting, offer no services for children. His focus for expansion is less on the number of clients served and more on the number of communities in which he can practice.

Currently, he sees 12 children and coleads three family sessions per week. His target market includes four towns with populations of under 1500.

Demographics

According to census and school-district data, there are approximately 600 potential clients (children between the ages of 2 and 18) in the communities that Max is targeting.

Competition

The psychiatric wing of the community hospital offers crisis intervention for children. That is the only direct competition that Max faces. The indirect competition, however, is immense. Much of the community expresses distrust of mental health professionals and the potential benefit their services provide. Consequently, Max's greatest competition is attitude.

MAX'S MARKETING OBJECTIVES

Max intends to provide direct service for children in four communities in addition to the one in which he resides. He plans to accomplish this goal in a one-year period.

MAX'S MARKETING STRATEGIES

Max's first task involves educating the communities in which he intends to practice about the value of his services. He has decided to approach the communities through the schools, physicians, churches, and childcare facilities. Here is his plan:

1. List the schools, churches, family practice physicians and childcare facilities in the four communities, by next week.
2. Develop by the end of next month a contact in each community who will make referrals and suggest other contacts.
3. Call and visit the contacts by the end of the quarter, asking each to arrange a speaking engagement/ demonstration at his or her facility.
4. At the speaking engagements, discuss child development, the use of art in wellness, and parent-child relations.
5. Also at speaking engagements, distribute cards on which participants write questions. Answer these at the talks and use them to develop future talks.
6. Offer to write a monthly column for the local newspapers. The same column could be used for several of the papers. Contact editors by next month.
7. Within two months of meeting with contacts, arrange a four-session group in each of the communities that focuses on "child-enrichment" for primary school age children.
8. Arrange a four-session parent-child group for preschool age children in each of the communities, within two months of the enrichment classes.

9. Document change in practice after completion of each step and at three-month intervals.

Discussion

A final word about marketing plans: use them as you would road maps on a journey across the U.S. No single map is sufficient for the entire trip. A general map of the U.S. may be sufficient to plan the interstate travel portion. You will need, however, detailed maps to explore major cities or to visit particular sights. You will also need various state maps to find your way on county and state roads. So, too, you will need various *maps* (marketing plans) to guide you on your professional *journey*. You may develop more general plans to guide you to two-year or five-year goals or during a certain stage of your life (for example, when your children are young). You may develop more specific plans to reach a particular group of potential patients or to market a particular aspect of your specialty. Creating marketing plans is a dynamic, ongoing process. As you, your community, and your field grow and change, so too should your marketing plans.

AREAS OF SPECIALIZATION

In our opinion, the decision to specialize has many advantages. The most obvious is that one usually chooses to specialize in areas in which one has expertise, that are enjoyable, and that produce the most positive results—in other words, areas in which the chances for therapeutic success are high. Specializing can also help you tailor your work schedule and environment. From a business perspective, the increasing competition demands a more targeted market. Specialization can focus your marketing effort and create a niche—that is, an area of practice where a very specific need exists in your market, which you can fill in a way that meets that specific need. Once established within this niche, you are likely to get more referrals from a greater variety of sources. The burgeoning field of chemical dependency counseling is a perfect example. From alcohol counseling came a model for other drug dependency counseling; from other drug dependency counseling came a model for codependency counseling. Clearly, too, the trend in contractual arrangements between independent practitioners and hospitals or health care plans decidedly favors specialization. (Chapter 5 discusses the relationship between the independent practitioner and hospitals/health care plans.)

Table 2 is a partial and personal list of specialties that we think are in demand now and show signs of remaining that way in the 1990s. Based on your own experience and that of your colleagues, you will probably be able to think of other specialties not listed here.

TABLE 2
Specialties

adult children of alcoholics
AIDS counseling
career counseling
chemical dependency
child sexual abuse therapy
child sexual assault prevention
codependency
counseling children of divorce
counseling gifted children
counseling infertile couples
displaced worker/relocation counseling
eating disorders
employee relations counseling
expressive arts therapy
geriatric counseling
grief counseling
organizational development
parenting skills
sex therapy
sexual addictions counseling
spirituality
sports psychology
women's issues

Once you have decided to specialize, you need to assess your skills, training, preferences, and the types of clients in your practice. You also need to examine the needs of your community. If this process sounds familiar, it is—it repeats basic marketing planning found earlier. Determine if your specialization requires additional training and/or certification or licensing. Several options are available for training: university and continuing education classes, reading materials, internships, workshops and seminars, certification programs, cofacilitation and supervision, and affiliation with professional organizations, hospitals, and mental health delivery systems (EAPs, PPOs, etc.). If your specialization encompasses a need that has been recently identified, your opportunities for training in traditional settings will likely be limited, and you will be best served by ferreting out those individuals already working in the area and reading as widely as possible in related areas. Although training may be more difficult to come by, you will be in a good position to market a specialty on the cutting edge of therapeutic practice.

A cautionary word about specialization: the therapist has a dual responsibility. On the one hand, the therapist should become familiar with a wide range of therapeutic modalities and topics, including those covered in the mass media. On the other hand, the therapist is required to represent his or her qualifications and knowledge accurately and without embellishment. Reading a couple of books does not constitute a specialization. You owe it to yourself and to your clients to take advantage of every opportunity to develop your specialty: reading, consultation, internships, continuing education classes, and so on.

CASE STUDIES—DEVELOPING A SPECIALTY

1. Sports Psychology

One of Ralph's specialty areas is sports psychology, which addresses issues specific to being an athlete. These issues may include performance anxiety, the role of competition, and family stresses resulting from name recognition, travel, off-season/in-season changes, contract negotiation, and mood fluctuations. Ralph offers such services as 1) life planning to help an athlete develop an identity outside sports; 2) seminars for those in particular sports that deal with issues specific to that sport; and 3) direct clinical services for families and individuals.

Ralph began focusing on sports psychology about 14 years ago when two well-known sports figures, Reggie Jackson and his agent, Gary Walker, both of whom he knew personally, asked him to provide help for some teammates. Under the auspices of the United Development Company, Jackson and Walker were offering a program called "Life Planning" for athletes, and they asked Ralph to assist them. Ralph realized that even though sports is a big industry, and that being able to handle moods, feelings, and problems is very important to an athlete's performance, the mental health field had for the most part ignored the area. Ralph also realized that (1) he personally enjoyed sports and interacting with athletes; and (2) his group practice already contained some therapists who specialized in areas, such as biofeedback and hypnosis, relevant to the practice of sports psychology.

The Phoenix area, where Ralph practices, is a sports center of sorts—a number of professional athletes make their homes there, and the city is host to multiple winter baseball teams and professional golf tournaments. Ralph contacted some coaches, whom he already knew in other contexts, to find out what they thought was needed and, in turn, talked to athletes themselves to assess what services would be most beneficial to them. He noticed many similarities between professional athletes and the high profile corporate and professional people with whom he had extensive experience. From this information, he devised programs and techniques to meet the needs he had identified. For example, he developed a three-hour seminar on identity issues, stressing the idea that an athlete is a person first who also happens to be an athlete. He put together a group for athletes that examined the challenges involved in dealing with the mood swings associated with the degree of performance. He met with individual and groups of athletes to help them deal with issues they faced as they finished college, went through the signing process, and became professionals.

Choosing to specialize in sports psychology, in addition to providing personally satisfying work, also helped Ralph build his practice and a national network. At the time, since so few people were specializing in the area, Ralph enjoyed little competition and very high visibility.

Ralph points out that learning about sports psychology has become more systematized as literature and training programs—including seminars, internships, and supervision—are now available. To break into the field now, he suggests getting to know colleagues who specialize in this area and meeting with athletic directors and coaches. Forming associations with high schools may provide valuable experience in the field before trying to practice at the college and professional levels. (And in some cases, high school athletes are now feeling the same pressures and confronting the same issues that college athletes of 10 to 15 years ago did.) Although subspecialties within the field of sports psychology have not yet developed, Ralph thinks this may change over the next decade. For example, some therapists work exclusively with Olympic athletes. Developing a subspecialty within sports psychology may leave you very well positioned for the 1990s.

2. Spirituality

A specialization in spirituality issues results more from developing a certain approach to therapy than from acquiring a discrete body of knowledge. Nevertheless, developing this specialty requires the practitioner to expand his or her therapeutic knowledge and techniques. Donald Hall, a psychologist in independent practice in Colorado Springs who also works with Ralph in Scottsdale, explains the issue in terms of client demand (Personal Communication, March 1989). A survey of religious beliefs, he said, found that 95 percent of Americans in the sample identified themselves as religious in some way. In times of crisis, many people tend to put even more emphasis on spirituality as a coping resource. According to Hall, "people are now less willing to 'split up' their treatment by allowing the therapist to disregard spiritual issues by saying, 'That's out of my province.' Clients do not want therapists to be 'valueless technicians.' They expect therapists to be human, not to the point of imposing their values, but at least allowing a full range of issues to be discussed instead of labeling any concern as 'out-of-bounds.' "

There are many reasons for this increased emphasis on spirituality, according to Hall. Spirituality and psychology often intersect on issues encompassing the meaning and purpose of life, such as values and ultimate questions. In addition to questions of meaning, religion and psychology are also related in the concepts of anxiety, guilt, and self-esteem. These concerns cannot readily be separated from their "treatment" bases in religious concepts, such as, for example, confession, repentance, forgiveness, and restitution. In the field of psychology, various individuals (Jung, Frankl, William James) and certain approaches (existential therapy, 12-step programs) have dealt with spiritual as well as religious issues, but for the most part therapists in the U.S. have embraced a scientific focus, dismissing spirituality as a concern because it cannot be quantified. Too often, says Hall, therapists have decided, "We shouldn't be trying to deal with these issues with our clients because we know too little." (Personal Communication, March 1989). But clients are facing a vast array and complexity of problems—with relationships, parenting, drugs, violence—and demanding that **every resource possible** be brought to bear on the problem. "People aren't waiting around for therapists to decide it's okay to explore the spiritual dimension of life" (Personal Communication, 1989).

Another reason for the increased emphasis on spirituality is that churches and synagogues have gotten too big to support individual pastoral care. Increasingly, ministers, priests, and rabbis are referring members of their congregations to practitioners in the community. And these clients come to the therapist with a strong spiritual orientation already in place, expecting a certain respect for this dimension of their lives as well.

Unfortunately, says Hall, schools lag behind in offering

therapists-in-training the resources to deal with spiritual issues. Even seminaries, in their pastoral counseling training, focus on psychology more than on the theological implications of psychology. Hall points out that the best opportunities for training in this area may occur at professional organizations' meetings and conventions, where interest groups meet to discuss spiritual issues, share experiences and skills, and often invite theologically oriented professionals in to discuss issues with them. (Such meetings could also be organized within your own community.) The therapist may also find some courses in pastoral counseling especially helpful, where certain issues such as bereavement counseling, may be treated from a faith as well as psychological perspective. Another way to acquire such knowledge and skills is to create opportunities for co-counseling and joint sessions with those who do pastoral counseling or other therapists with experience and expertise in dealing with spiritual issues.

3. Childhood Trauma

"At this point, many people who choose this specialty are coming to it from their own victimization," according to Marilyn Murray, a specialist in the area of childhood trauma recovery (Personal Communication, April 1989). Murray defines the area as incorporating the wide range of physical, emotional, and sexual abuse that results in long-term difficulties for the individual.

Murray believes that it is not necessary to have been victimized to effectively treat those who have, but she is adamant that practitioners with this history "should not be doing counseling until they've worked through the issue in their own therapy. Those who haven't will be dealing with the sobbing child within themselves who will create problems not only for them but for their clients" (Personal Communication, April 1989). While that is a maxim preached to all therapists, regardless of history or area of practice, Murray believes that it is especially important in the context of trauma counseling.

Murray, who has earned a national reputation for her expertise in the field, asserts that therapists who specialize in working with adult survivors of childhood trauma will have entered a specialty that serves what she sees as "the greatest need." Media attention to child sexual assault has caused countless adults to begin to confront the histories they had repressed or minimized. According to Murray, these individuals are seeking help but are frustrated in their search to find therapists who are sufficiently knowledgeable in the area.

As far as Murray knows, no college or university offers a comprehensive course of study leading to a specialization in childhood trauma recovery. Thus, few researchers are involved in the work required to generate a theoretical base that might lead to curricular institutionalization. Further, although some therapists are experienced in working with survivors, the lack of theory leads to treatment that is often at best experimental and at worst counterproductive.

To specialize in childhood trauma recovery, Murray offers several suggestions to the clinician. First, develop an openness to whatever abuse issues may exist for you, however minimal. Second, take advantage of the myriad of relevant conferences and workshops, especially those that provide theory-based practice techniques. Third, read extensively but critically. You need to develop a discerning eye based on your and your clients' experiences and values. Fourth, if you are specializing in sexual abuse, get involved in crisis center counseling services that are available in your area. Most offer training programs for volunteers in which you can participate. They also offer groups for adults who were molested as children. These programs serve a variety of clients and are often clearinghouses for the most recent information in the field. If you become a volunteer and develop professional relationships with the staff, these programs also serve as excellent referral sources.

Murray adds that some of the most knowledgeable clinicians are the "front-liners," that is, those with other than Ph.D. or M.D. degrees but who have the most direct experience. She suggests you arrange to consult or work closely with them.

Jeff Kirkendall agrees with Murray that volunteering or working in a social service agency is vital to specializing in the area of sexual abuse counseling (Personal Communication, December 1989). Jeff Kirkendall and Carol Jarvis Kirkendall are a husband and wife therapy team specializing in the treatment of sexual abuse victims and perpetrators. They are also the authors of *Without Consent: How to Overcome Childhood Sexual Abuse.* In 1980, before they knew one another, Carol was the clinical director of the Center Against Sexual Assault in the Phoenix area, which at the time was the largest private, nonprofit center for sexual abuse treatment in the U.S. Jeff, who had just finished his master's degree, applied to the Center in response to a job opening. Although he was underqualified for the job, he began volunteering as a counselor because he realized that the experience would be important to his future employment and because he had been told that staff often look at the volunteer pool first when there are job openings.

Jeff says that working in a social service agency gave him the opportunity to try a number of different approaches to treatment and allowed him practical experience. He decided to specialize in sexual abuse therapy because he found the field personally challenging, though somewhat frightening too. The choice had a spiritual dimension for him as well in that, in dealing with both the victims and perpetrators of abuse, he felt called upon to address basic issues of the meaning and purpose of life and the role of evil. He contrasted his reasons with those of Carol, who chose to specialize in the field because she herself had been the victim of childhood abuse and wanted to use her experience to create something positive.

Jeff points out that working in an agency also helped both him and Carol identify numerous resources and develop credibility in the community (Personal Communication, December 1989). When they decided to enter independent practice in 1983, a large majority of their referrals came from people in probation and parole, judges, police departments, DES (Department of Economic Security) personnel, and other therapists with whom Jeff and Carol had worked when they were at the Center. For the first two to three years of their practice, because this referral base was so strong and because there were only about two or three other therapists in the valley specializing in sexual abuse, they did very little marketing.

With their decision to write a book about sexual abuse, Jeff and Carol began to cut back severely on the number of clients they were treating. When they finished the book a few years later, they realized they would have to concentrate on marketing their practice all over again. They discovered that a number of people had simply assumed they were no longer practicing—out of sight, out of mind. Further, they found the marketplace changed. The number of therapists specializing in sexual abuse had skyrocketed.

Jeff and Carol have now developed a marketing strategy designed to strengthen their practice and establish ties with institutions that can provide referrals. One important source of referrals is the 12-step programs. The Kirkendalls have found that once people deal with their substance addictions, they often discover issues of child abuse, neglect, and abandonment underlying their addictions. The Kirkendalls are also working to publicize their book. Ironically, the book is proving to be a good networking and marketing tool, even though the writing of it took a high toll on their practice.

Finally, Jeff and Carol are taking their practice in new directions. While they are still doing sexual abuse therapy, they are also becoming more diversified. At this writing, they are in the process of opening a second office in Payson, Arizona, which is in the Mogollon Rim area. They want to conduct day-long or overnight retreats into the rim country, which will holistically integrate consideration of nature and the environment with more traditional therapeutic and relationship issues.

If You Are Just Starting Out

We think it is important to add to our discussion of representative specialties a word about the relationship of specialization to the beginning independent practitioner. At the time of this writing, Marcus Earle, a certified psychologist and Ralph's son, had been in independent practice for about a year and a half. He thinks it is extremely important to establish himself as a specialist (Personal Communication, December 1989). He graduated with a Ph.D. in marriage and family therapy, which he thought would provide a distinct and marketable specialization. Unfortunately, he discovered that this alone did not make him stand out from his colleagues or from institutions such as hospitals. He then decided to focus on his expertise in chemical dependency, and he combined this with marriage and family therapy. Again, though, he found himself in a very large pool of established practitioners where he did not particularly stand out.

About this time, Ralph and a colleague were working on a book about sexual addictions. Marcus realized that his background in addictions therapy had prepared him to work with his father and his father's colleague in this area. So he began to read journals and books and attend workshops and seminars focused on sexual addiction. Soon, he was able to develop talks he could present to various audiences—church groups, community organizations, hospitals. He volunteered to speak about the subject on radio and TV news and special report programming. This specialization in sexual addictions treatment is now giving Marcus an "identity" in the community that he can market.

Marcus Earle emphasizes how frustratingly slow and difficult the processes of marketing a specialization and developing an independent practice are, even with the entré he had because of Ralph's work and the public focus on sexual addictions. In retrospect, Marcus thinks it is important for those in school to begin to develop a specialty by focusing their research, papers, clinical training, and so on, on a particular area. By their very nature, educational programs will provide the general, well-rounded background a therapist needs, but he says it is up to the student to seek out a specialty. He recommends reading widely in professional journals and topical books and searching oneself in order to identify one's own interests. Although it is useful to be aware of areas of greatest demand and popular interest, he thinks that in the end personal interest and excitement about a particular specialty are the best guides to choosing a specialty. At the same time, he fully expects to expand his specialty areas over time as he develops new interests and identifies new needs.

If You Are In Mid-Stream

We would like to reiterate Marcus Earle's idea of growth and development in the process of specializing. The experience of Brady Wilson, a psychologist in independent practice in Scottsdale, illuminates the kinds of changes an independent practitioner may experience throughout the course of his or her career (Personal Communication, December 1989). Wilson has been in independent practice for over a decade. He originally began his practice working with children. After a few years, he realized he was facing some major marketing challenges: first, his practice was almost completely dependent on indirect referrals (children rarely refer!) and, second, schools and physicians were becoming increasingly conservative about referring to independent practitioners. So Wilson expanded his practice and became a kind of "family practice" psychologist. This strategy was fruitful for a time, but then, in examining his business records, he noted that his insurance reimbursements had fallen from 70 percent of gross receipts to 30 percent. From his referral records, Wilson knew his referrals had been increasing astronomically, but people were not following up on the referrals because, for example, Wilson was not on their PPO list or they were members of an HMO—in short, insurance reimbursements were becoming harder and harder to come by.

During this same period, Wilson had been working occasionally with a plaintiff employee attorney who specialized in wrongful discharge and sexual harassment suits. Wilson began doing evaluation work for some of the attorney's court cases and proceeded to provide therapy focused on *workplace trauma* for some of the attorney's clients. Wilson started by focusing on the grief and loss issues involved in the workplace situation. He soon realized that issues beyond grief and loss were involved. He began reading everything he could in related areas. Although some theoretical work has been done in the area of sexual harassment, very little work has been done in the general area of workplace trauma. Wilson began to focus on this area to develop both treatment methods and theoretical models. As he gained further expertise in this area, he began to publish a quarterly newsletter, which is sent to plaintiff employee lawyers and defense attorneys specializing in labor law. He now works with about 40 lawyers. In addition to evaluation and therapy, he also consults with attorneys and engages in deposition and expert witness work. Wilson envisions his next step as consulting with corporations to train management in effective policy implementation so as to avoid litigation for wrongful termination. Eventually Wilson hopes to establish a foundation that would disseminate information, support research, and assist employees in issues related to workplace trauma.

We think Brady Wilson's career is a good example of the kind of evolution an independent practice can undergo. This evolution involves a constant dialogue between therapeutic and business interests and often results in changes in a therapist's area of specialization. Wilson repeated a conversation that had had a profound effect on him (Personal Communication, December 1989). When he was trying to figure out how to improve his practice, he spoke to a friend who worked in the corporate world. Wilson asked her what corporations do when their product is not moving or is otherwise faltering. What they generally do, she replied, is to make the mistake of trying harder to do the same thing. What they do not typically do is to try something innovative, or creative, or different.

Developing an area of specialization requires the same creativity and innovation necessary to build and maintain an independent practice in general. It is not something you do once and then forget about. Even if you stay in the same general field throughout your career, in order to keep your practice flourishing and yourself fully engaged, you will have to remain open to the evolutionary possibilities that present themselves.

5/
From Contact to Contract: Institutional Affiliation

You now have some good ideas about how to take your *private* practice public, thus creating an *independent* practice. You may, however, begin to wonder about maintaining your independence in the face of burgeoning megainstitutions, which now provide an ever-increasing percentage of health care services in this country. Although these are not all large organizations, the trend is toward consolidation.

Given this fact, it is unrealistic to think you can develop a successful independent practice without having some level of affiliation with institutions—for example, universities, hospitals, clinics, or health care corporations. Furthermore, there are definite advantages to affiliating with institutions. Perhaps the most obvious advantage is that marketing and building a practice are far easier when you have access to the large clientele these institutions represent. Hospitals often serve as referral hubs in an area, both in direct referral of their outpatient clients and by referral from staff clinicians who have become part of your professional network.

Cross-marketing (see p. 64) with an institution provides you with referrals and name recognition; in other words, you become the beneficiary of the marketing, advertising, and public relations efforts of the institution. For example, Community Hospital advertises in the local paper that Dr. Famous will give a workshop and sell copies of her most recent book. The hospital and Dr. Famous have shared the cost of advertising, and both will benefit from the connection. Hospitals are also in a good position to provide you with an overview of clinical and marketing trends in mental health care. Other advantages include educational opportunities through in-services, access to team therapy, and concomitant clinical feedback. The decision then is not so much whether or not to affiliate, but how.

Nevertheless, many independent practitioners fear that affiliation will result in the loss of autonomy that they sought in the first place by becoming independent practitioners. These fears are sometimes supported by reality. Some practitioners are exploited to such an extent that they are unable to sustain their own practices. For instance, an institution may require so substantial a time commitment that the practitioner cannot or does not sufficiently market the nonaffiliated portion of the practice. Additionally, some practitioners have suffered from *guilt by association* if the institution develops a less-than-stellar reputation.

Falling prey to the disadvantages can, however, be mitigated by remembering that affiliation should be *mutually* beneficial. The institution receives the benefit of your knowledge of the needs and attitudes of your community, your professional expertise, and the marketing of your reputation without having to provide you with employee benefits. Too often, however, private practitioners forget the value they bring to the institution. They tend to approach the institution in an obsequious manner because they diminish their own professional value and potential contribution. (Unfortunately, the bureaucracy inherent to institutions sometimes reinforces this perceived inequality.)

Moving from contact to contract involves three major steps: market planning (once again), negotiation-contract, and implementation. Two-thirds of this process, you will notice, revolve around business skills rather than therapeutic skills—with good reason. Dealing with highly structured corporations requires access to either your own or an advisor's business expertise. In this context, business naiveté can seriously compromise your practice.

MARKET PLANNING

To create an effective affiliation, the first step is to assess the marketplace. This time the market consists of two types of institutions: mental health facilities (hospitals, clinics, etc.) and mental health components of health care organizations such as HMOs, PPOs, and EAPs. When you were doing your marketing plan in Chapter 4, you probably included an analysis of the institutional market. Because your analysis was not specifically focused on institutions alone, you may have some gaps in your information about them. According to Karen Wiese, administrator of Desert Hills Residential Treatment Center and Hospital in Tucson, practitioners should evaluate a hospital facility according to the following criteria (Personal Communication, April 1989):

1. *Program Innovation.* Does the facility provide a creative environment? Flexibility in both program design and scheduling? Is it willing to support new programs or new approaches to existing ones?
2. *Financial Stability.* What is the longevity of programs? Have programs been discontinued from lack of funding? What is the rate of staff turnovers and layoffs?
3. *Cotherapy Philosophy.* What are the opportunities and restrictions?
4. *Open Staff Policy.* Try to affiliate with a facility that has an open staff policy, that is, one which does not restrict treatment privileges to its employees or a limited number of outside practitioners, and that does not restrict privileges based on education other than the hospital's basic credentialing requirements.
5. *Joint Commission Accreditation.* This is the only nationwide accrediting agency; it evaluates a facility's quality of care every three years.
6. *Educational Opportunities.* What opportunities will I have to develop my skills or increase my knowledge? How will these contribute to my long-range plans?

7. *Marketing Program.* How much does the facility spend on marketing? What percentage of its total budget does this amount represent? For what activities are marketing dollars spent? Wiese believes that excessive and/or sensationalized advertising is a waste of money and represents a "flash in the pan" approach as opposed to a longer-term commitment that emphasizes referral development and community education.

8. *Financial Policy Regarding Admissions and Insurance.* Financial policy can affect the therapist's reimbursement. Some hospitals do not require patients to document coverage. Unpaid patient bills can mean unreimbursed therapists. Some hospitals will provide a patient referred by an independent practitioner with a free bed; in return, practitioners try to limit the number of incidences where this is required by attending to a patient's financial status before referral and admittance.

9. *Hospital Administration.* Is the administration visible in the community and committed to building referrals? Is the administration sensitive to community and clinician need?

10. *Programming.* Is the facility committed to looking for opportunities for growth based on community need and staff creativity?

11. *Mechanisms for Fostering Clinician's Involvement.* Has the facility taken steps to insure the smooth functioning of its clinician credentialing process? Does the hospital regularly invite clinicians to determine their level of involvement with hospitalized patients? Does the hospital support the level of patient involvement chosen by clinicians?

Your goal is to select an affiliation that best matches your personality and your patients' needs, as well as one that fosters direct communication between you and the institutional staff.

Part of your information-gathering procedure is to assess your appropriateness to the institutional market. Wiese looks for the following qualities in clinicians:

1. *Entrepreneurial Enthusiasm.* The hospital looks for clinicians who exhibit enthusiasm and commitment through comments such as "I can offer your patients . . . ," "I'd love to do an in-service on . . . ," "Let's do a seminar for the community on. . . ."
2. *Ability To Work Responsibly as a Team Member.* Hospital programs involve input from many sources about treatment. They frequently expect outside clinicians to value and incorporate this input and to report clinical findings back to the team.
3. *Treatment Philosophy Consistent with an Inpatient Option.* Therapists who solicit hospital affiliation but decry hospitalizing their clients do not endear themselves to hospital staff members.
4. *Credentials/Experience Commensurate with the Institution's Therapeutic and Marketing Goals.*

Once you have determined the feasibility of a relationship with a particular institution or program, you can then decide the specific service you wish to offer and then position yourself to create the liaisons just as you planned in Chapter 4.

NEGOTIATION/CONTRACT

As in any business transaction—from setting a client's fee to closing a contract with a major HMO—negotiation is inevitable. The most appropriate stance in these negotiations is *win-win*, that is, a negotiation in which the interests of both parties are integrated into the final outcome. However, assume that the burden of responsibility for a win-win interaction rests with you. This does not preclude fairmindedness by the institution.

Win-win negotiations require you to employ many of your therapeutic skills, but to a different purpose. The intended outcome is a mutually beneficial contract rather than amelioration of psychopathology. You will need to listen actively,

TABLE 3
Guidelines for Negotiation*

Problem   **Solution**
Positional Bargaining: Which Game Should   *Change the Game—*
You Play?   *Negotiate on the*
                                                      Merits

Soft	**Hard**	**Principled**
Partipants are friends.	Participants are adversaries.	Participants are problem-solvers.
The goal is agreement.	The goal is victory.	The goal is a wise outcome reached efficiently and amicably.
Make concessions to cultivate the relationship.	Demand concessions as a condition of the relationship.	Separate the people from the problem.
Be soft on the people and the problem.	Be hard on the problem and the people.	Be soft on the people, hard on the problem.
Trust others.	Distrust others.	Proceed independent of trust.
Change your position easily.	Dig in to your position.	Focus on interests, not positions.
Make offers.	Make threats.	Explore interests.
Disclose your bottom line.	Mislead as to your bottom line.	Avoid having a bottom line.
Accept one-sided losses to reach agreement.	Demand one-sided gains as the price of agreement.	Invent options for mutual gain.
Search for the single answer: the one *they* will accept.	Search for the single answer: the one *you* will accept.	Develop multiple options to choose from; decide later.
Insist on agreement.	Insist on your position.	Insist on using objective criteria.
Try to avoid a contest of will.	Try to win a contest of will.	Try to reach a result based on standards independent of will.
Yield to pressure.	Apply pressure.	Reason and be open to reasons; yield to principle, not pressure.

*Reprinted with permission from Fisher and Ury, 1983, p. 13.

evaluate the communication process, respect yourself as well as those with whom you are negotiating, be clear, and be honest. Several texts produced by the business community describe win-win negotiations in detail. *Getting to Yes* by Roger Fisher and William Ury of the Harvard Negotiation Project details effective negotiation strategies that invite participants to be problem solvers rather than "I win, you lose" (hard) or "You win, I lose" (soft) tacticians. Table 3 provides guidelines for negotiation.

IMPLEMENTATION

Implementation is a two-step process. The first is the obvious carrying out of the services for which you have been contracted. The second process actually consists of analyzing and positioning yourself to receive additional contract opportunities, that is, repeating the market analysis and negotiation process. As you become more familiar with the institution, you are in a better position to know the gaps in its services and the areas in which they intend to develop. Once inside the workings of the hospital or institution, you can suggest areas where you can fill its needs and become an active participant in strategic planning.

Of all the steps involved in affiliation, implementation is the most individualized. The following case study illustrates the complexity and rewards of affiliating with a larger entity.

In 1988, Joan and three of her colleagues were awarded a significant contract to provide a range of employee assistance program (EAP) services for a major employer. Her experience illuminates both the process of getting the contract and the possibilities for continuous marketing and growth:

Unlike most contract negotiations, these began when the company— call it Verylarge Company—issued an RFP (request for proposal) to provide EAP services and asked me to respond. They indicated they were dissatisfied with their current EAP provider.

In the past, several of their employees had been my clients, and the company had referred employees to me for assessment, so the company was familiar with my work. I identified three colleagues who I thought would be competent, ethical, and fun to work with. Two of these people also had extensive experience setting up and managing EAPs. I could expect these two to possibly be competitors in the future, so it made sense to ally with them. The four of us comprised the management team and owned the EAP.

I sat down with representatives from Verylarge to see what their needs were. We began by providing the basic EAP services (assessment, referral, case management). We were adamant about providing the highest quality, most efficient service—in the most cost-effective way.

In the first months, three of us carried beepers and gave the number to the EAP contact within Verylarge. Even though local hospitals were willing to cover emergencies for us, we preferred to maintain control over and consistency of service. The company was very impressed. We maintained frequent contact with Verylarge and gradually saw an opportunity to expand our services. Our contract now includes management consulting and organizational development; third-party administration of benefits; preemployment/ promotion assessment screening; preventive (and legal) chemical dependency screening and assessment; human resource development; and supervisor training. Because of the reputation we have acquired from this work, other companies are now coming to us and requesting similar programs. Furthermore, companies whom we solicit are more willing to consider our program because of our success with Verylarge.

Harry Saslow, Ph.D. is a partner in Joan's EAP team. In his opinion (Personal Communication, March 1989), the main reason Verylarge first approached Joan was her "high visibility in this community." He added that his interest in pursuing the contract was based on the potential opportunity for work in areas other than the basic EAP services. "EAP services are similar to those given by Boy Scouts with first-aid credentials. They help people over the mild hump and are crisis-oriented." However, once affiliated with Verylarge, the team saw ways to be more valuable to the staff and management. "The services we have developed can be classified as risk management. They are highly beneficial and interesting to offer—and we do this for a fine fee, more like a retainer than a capitation" [fee-per-client].

RELEARNING YOUR ABCs—A PRIMER OF ORGANIZATIONAL HEALTH CARE

Most practitioners have had some experience affiliating, usually with hospitals, clinics, or social service agencies. Based on our experience and that of many of our colleagues, we believe that health maintenance organizations, employee assistance plans, and preferred provider organizations, as well as variations on these three structures, form an increasingly

---

TABLE 4
ABCs of Health Care*

Copayment: Out-of-pocket cost to the consumer.

Employee Assistance Program (EAP): Programs designed to deal with problems in the workplace that may diminish productivity; may be internal or external.

Exclusive Provider Organizations (EPO): A hybrid between a PPO and an HMO; created by self-insured companies for their employees; restrictions similar to HMO.

Exclusion: Medical condition or type of treatment not covered by plan. Some plans exclude mental health treatment.

Health Maintenance Organization (HMO): Provides prepaid services to members with minimal copayment; some structured on wellness model; members must usually use plan facilities and providers.

Indemnity Plan: New name for major medical insurance.

IPA: Variously interpreted as Independent Provider Association, Independent Physician Association, and Individual Practice Associations. Like HMOs, lower-cost, prepaid health plans with fixed charge for members and limits for number of therapy sessions; unlike HMOs, members go to provider's office; also can refer to an organization of providers formed to negotiate contracts with HMOs, PPOs, hospitals, and so on.

Preferred Provider Organization (PPO): Group of providers with whom employers, insurance companies, or other third-party payers contract; paid fee-for-service at a lower rate.

---

*Adapted with permission from Adams, 1987, p. 24, and D'Andrea, 1988, p. 77.

lucrative market. Because mental health care delivery has become so diverse, understanding the variety of structures, and how to operate effectively within them, allows the independent practitioner more flexibility in tailoring a practice. The downside of this diversity and growth, however, is the instability of the industry. The consensus of those who monitor health care delivery trends is that the movement toward alternative delivery and financing of health care is permanent, but the structures remain in flux. Consequently, our suggestions for evaluating your potential relationship with these structures are offered as broad guidelines for you to adapt to the situation in your community.

The change in delivery of services is based on the key concept of *managed mental health care*. This concept can be understood in two ways: 1) financially, it refers to a strategy of predetermining cost limitations for services; 2) clinically, it refers to an approach to therapy emphasizing brief outpatient care. All of the alternative delivery systems that we discuss are variations of this basic concept. Each system has its own focus but none is inherently superior to the others.

Employee Assistance Programs (EAPs)

George Watkins, publisher of the *EAP Digest* and the *Student Assistance Journal* and president of Performance Resource Press, defines an EAP as "a company-based program for purposes of identifying [and treating] problems affecting job performance" (Personal Communication, March 1989). An EAP program can be internal or external. Internal programs, usually limited to very large companies, hire their own clinicians; external programs refer clients to outside clinicians. Contracts are made either with a vendor who subcontracts clinicians or with individual clinicians. Clinicians, although not necessarily members of the same group practice, are designated by the company as a preferred provider organization (PPO). According to Watkins, many practitioners misunderstand EAPs. "They come to me and say they want to be an EAP. But they don't. What they want is to contract their treatment services to the company or to an EAP vendor" (Personal Communication, March 1989).

According to George Vroom, a marriage and family therapist in independent practice and director of DVS Associates—a consulting group for EAPs and corporations—EAPs began in the effort to cut health care costs and at the same time respond to the diminished productivity and increasing absenteeism resulting from chemical dependency among employees (Personal Communication, March 1989). The focus of EAPs soon expanded to include treatment for depression and family problems, because these too have a profound impact on productivity and attendance. Companies saw the EAP as an effective means to reduce employee turnover.

EAP vendors serve as brokers between the company and the independent clinician. Vroom describes EAP vendors as "conduits" between the corporate and therapeutic worlds (Personal Communication, March 1989). The choice to become a vendor should emerge after a practitioner has cultivated relationships with respected colleagues and corporate decision-makers. Typically, a vendor is an independent contractor who provides assessment, referral, and case management services for the company, as well as brief therapy (on the average, up to eight sessions); those clients who require longer-term therapy are referred. Brokers are usually paid by capitation (that is, a fee per employee based on the total number of employees in the company). At the point of referral to a longer-term primary therapist, payment is assumed by the company's insurance. Watkins notes that in the long-term, EAP vendors may become primary or preferred providers rather than just brokers for those services (Personal Communication, March 1989).

Those who are considering offering EAP services may want to explore the possibility of becoming EAP vendors. There are no licenses required; however, Watkins recommends specialized EAP training to become a vendor/broker. It is a matter of determining company needs in your community and assembling a team to fill them. If you have no experience working with EAPs, be sure to incorporate into your network individuals who do.

Watkins predicts that more and more companies, even large companies that have traditionally established in-house programs, will engage external vendors in the future because they often prove to be more cost effective and better able to maintain confidentiality (Personal Communication, March 1989). He adds that a company manager, hired to oversee services, will be the only vestige of the in-house EAP program. The manager will refer employees to the contracted broker. Thus, Watkins encourages independent practitioners to get to know the EAP brokers with large contracts in their communities.

Watkins suggests analyzing your revenue sources to determine whether your practice would benefit from pursuing EAP affiliation (Personal Communication, March 1989). In general, the benefits of EAP affiliation are directly proportional to the percentage of revenue that comes from third-party payments. In other words, assume your payments are 25 percent from HMOs, 25 percent from clients, and 50 percent from third parties (insurance companies). In Watkins's construction, because half of your collections come from third-party payment, your practice is likely to suffer in the near future unless you replace at least part of that 50 percent with payment from other sources—such as EAPs. Insurance companies are gradually moving to PPOs; therefore, third-party payment will become less available to the individual practitioner. At the same time, employers are mandating that their employees use EAP-type mental health services. Thus, the unaffiliated independent practitioner will have access to less of the potential client population and a lower level of reimbursement (Personal Communication, March 1989).

If you choose to pursue EAP affiliation, Watkins identifies three factors that will enhance your chances of securing EAP contracts (Personal Communication, March 1989). First, and most important, is your reputation for ethical and competent practice; your references should support your reputation. Second, you must be willing to work with the EAP, that is, be a team player and effective communicator. Like family systems therapy, treatment of an employee involves consideration of the client's interaction with company culture and fellow employees. The EAP and the company it represents as well as the client/employee are all your clients. Watkins warns, "If you don't like to be questioned about your methods (diagnostic and therapeutic), don't go into EAP work" (Personal Communication, March 1989). Finally, EAPs seek clinicians with specific credentials. Watkins advises clinicians to have at least a master's degree (MSW, MA, and Ph.D. degrees are most commonly accepted) (Personal Communication, March 1989). Specialty training in the field of chemical dependency as well as certification in this area is helpful. Other certifications that may be useful include Certified Employee Assistance Professional (CEAP) and Certified Social Worker (CSW). Involvement in relevant professional associations such as ALMACA or EASNA (Employee Assistance Society of North America) is useful as an expression of good faith and interest in the field (though not of experience/expertise). Vroom warns, however, that EAP recruitment at professional meetings is diminishing because practitioners' solicitation for contracts has in some cases overwhelmed EAP representatives (Personal Communication, March 1989).

In addition to your personal qualities, the organization of your practice may be relevant. Watkins conjectures that EAPs may have some preference for working with solo practitioners or small groups rather than large groups because, in the EAP's perception, it is able to retain more control and accessibility and command more accountability (Personal Communication, March 1989). This advantage is particularly noticeable in *assessment* contracts; however, a large group may have an advantage in contracting for *treatment* services because it is able to offer a wider range of skills and areas of expertise than an individual or small group can.

Competition for EAP-related work is increasing, primarily because EAP pay-scales tend to be significantly higher. Watkins notes that an MA counselor with three to five years' experience may earn approximately twice as much as an EAP manager than he or she would as an independent practitioner (Personal Communication, March 1989). Graduate programs are more aggressively pursuing placement in EAPs for their graduates; however, says Watkins, "workplace knowledge is critical. The therapist needs to know about corporate culture.

Someone with experience in a corporate setting would be more attractive than a new graduate" (Personal Communication, March 1989). Vroom believes that many practitioners are drawn to EAPs with the expectation of referrals to their independent practices (Personal Communication, March 1989). While referrals (and marketing opportunities) do result, Vroom cautions that EAP work is not a "gold mine," and in fact the practitioner should be prepared for occasional pro bono work for company employees.

If you decide to offer EAP services, you must then decide in what capacity: you can provide clinical and/or brokering services. According to Watkins, in whatever capacity you affiliate with a company, you should look for a company that

1. Has an EAP policy and procedures manual for clinicians. Often this has not yet been developed, allowing you the chance to influence policies and procedures;
2. Gives you access to the worksite in order to better understand corporate culture;
3. Invites you to initiate educational programs for employees (stress reduction, weight control, smoking cessation); and
4. Has a company policy statement prior to establishing an EAP. This statement delineates the company's philosophy about helping employees deal with personal problems. It reassures the employee that seeking help will not affect opportunities for promotion and salary increases and that covered costs will indeed be borne by the employer. It also warns the employee that seeking help will not exempt him or her from standard disciplinary procedures (Personal Communication, March 1989).

Health Maintenance Organizations (HMOs)

HMOs are independent companies that hire staff and establish facilities to provide a variety of health care services to their patients/members at a cost below that of traditional delivery systems. Membership costs are based on a flat rate per member and are prepaid, usually by an employer. Employees/patients pay a token membership fee per paycheck and a small copayment at the time of service. The HMO covers services provided by its staff in its facilities; it may also cover, at least in part, emergency services sought by members traveling outside the service area.

HMOs were devised based on two premises: a wellness, preventive approach to health care, and cost-containment of medical care based on a treatment philosophy of limited intervention. Most HMOs limit the number of therapy sessions they will cover—usually 20. Again, as with EAPs, the emphasis is on brief therapy.

For the independent practitioner seeking part-time agency employment, the HMO may provide many opportunities. If you are just beginning to practice, for example, working for an HMO may allow you to make connections and build a network in the community in anticipation of starting your own independent practice. An HMO offers little opportunity to those who solely want to practice independently unless you affiliate with a PPO or IPA, for example, that in turn contracts with an HMO. For that reason, we do not treat affiliation in detail, though the principles are similar to those for PPO affiliation. The criteria for seeking hospital affiliation provided earlier in this chapter will also be helpful in seeking HMO employment.

Preferred Provider Organizations (PPOs)

At the time of this writing, PPOs are the fastest growing segment of health care delivery systems (Adams, 1987). In theory, a PPO is a contractual agreement in which providers— therapists, physicians, hospitals—"agree to render a specified range of health care services to a purchaser, such as a union [or a company or an insurance plan], at a rate of reimbursement below the norm. The idea is to guarantee a referral base of clients by charging a lower fee" (Adams, 1987, p. 25). In fact, according to John M. Thomas, senior vice president for Preferred Health Care Limited, which owns the largest psychiatric PPO in the U.S., PPOs vary widely because they are legally defined on a state by state basis relative to such factors as standard insurance plans within a particular state (Personal Communication, April 1989).

PPOs differ from HMOs in that PPOs can contract providers from a variety of sources—for example, individual practitioners, group practices, or hospitals. These providers are independent contractors, not employees as in an HMO arrangement. In a PPO, providers are paid fee-for-service; in an HMO, providers are salaried regardless of services provided, though the most productive members may be rewarded with higher salaries and/or bonuses. The purchaser of PPO services pays a monthly fee, the client may also pay a small monthly fee, and the client also pays a copayment at the time of service. The PPO does not own the service facility. If a client needs to be referred to a specialist, both PPOs and HMOs generally expect the referral to be to a practitioner within the service organization.

Related to the PPO is the EPO or Exclusive Provider Organization. These are most often formed by very large companies that are self-insured (that is, employees are covered by the company's own funds and the employer, not an insurance company, assumes all the risk). Thomas notes that such EPOs, because they are exempt from certain state laws (the result of E.R.I.S.A., a federal regulation overriding state laws), have much more flexibility than PPOs in determining whom they will accept as a preferred provider (individual or group) (Personal Communication, April 1989). For this reason, Thomas urges independent practitioners to educate themselves about EPOs in their geographic area.

Therapists are organizing or joining PPOs in greater numbers to preserve at least some of their autonomy in the face of ever more common mergers that create health care conglomerates. In Thomas's opinion, the advantages of affiliation with PPOs will grow more pronounced in the future because he sees companies moving away from traditional indemnity plans and HMOs to contract with PPOs as their major providers (Personal Communication, April 1989). On the other hand, he points out, a PPO puts its contracted providers at a disadvantage because of its lower *per unit* price. However, what the practitioner loses in reimbursement per patient may be compensated for in greater client volume. Offering a wider range of services, which can generate clients from a variety of sources, may also make up the discrepancy.

As we have pointed out in our discussion of other kinds of affiliation, there are certain characteristics that PPOs will look for in their providers (or purchasers will look for in their PPOs). Thomas's advice for independent practitioners seeking to establish or affiliate with a PPO incorporates both what the organizations look for and the steps for best positioning yourself for PPO establishment or affiliation (Personal Communication, April 1989):

1. Find out what credentials are required to be part of a PPO. These are determined by individual states.
2. Become familiar with EPOs and major insurers in your geographic area.
3. Develop a specialized niche—do something no one else is doing, or do it in a different way—in your geographic area.
4. Find a way to prove you have a better mousetrap. An example: Deal with psychiatric workers' compensation issues in such a way as to return the workers to work more quickly and at a higher functional level. Many would-be providers have developed pilot programs and used them to interest self-insured companies in a wider range of services.
5. Become a hub for independent practitioners in your community. Develop linkages with individuals, groups, and/or institutions that provide various levels of care and kinds of services. The more formal these linkages are—contracts, letters of agreement, etc.—the more persuasive they are.

On the other side, what should you as an independent practitioner look for in a PPO? Thomas advises practitioners to consider the following factors (Personal Communication, April 1989):

1. *Reimbursement Levels.* Even though PPOs reimburse at a lower rate than indemnity programs, not all PPOs reimburse at the same level.
2. *Referral Process.* From where do referrals come? How many referrals and of what kind will you be getting? Look for PPOs that *proactively triage*, which means that the PPO has set up in advance methods to refer clients based on need to therapists best suited to meet those needs based on skill and experience.
3. *Size.* A very large PPO may not provide you with sufficient referrals to be worthwhile.
4. *Exclusivity.* Just because a PPO calls itself a PPO does not necessarily mean it is one. Some PPOs include everyone in the universe on their list, mitigating against their stated purpose of guaranteeing a certain level of referrals.
5. *Provider Selection Process.* How carefully does the PPO scrutinize its providers? Being associated with a PPO that does not screen its providers carefully can cause serious problems for you. For example, you do not want to rely on a psychiatrist who has been involved in unethical activity to prescribe for your patients.

It is possible to be an independent practitioner and maintain the autonomy that attracted you to this form of practice. However, to do so you will need to monitor the systems of health care nationally and locally. These institutions are not threats but rather can be seen as opportunities for the practitioner who is positioned to effectively use them.

PART III
Professional Identity

6/
Soloist or Symphony: Structuring Your Business

WHAT KIND OF PRACTICE?

More and more, group practice of one type or another is becoming the norm, but opportunities for solo practice will still be available in the 1990s. Our experience, personalities, and our perceptions of clients' needs have led us to prefer a group structure; not all independent practitioners will come to the same choice. The notion of group *versus* solo practice is misleading. There are numerous arrangements that combine elements of group and solo practice. While the terms "group" and "solo" sound clearcut, in fact, they can be ambiguous. (They also should not be considered synonymous with the legal structures "sole proprietorship" and "partnership" or "corporation.") A solo practice is obviously a single person practicing alone; however, the solo practitioner might share office space and consult with two other therapists. A PPO may look like a group practice but in fact consists of a collection of solo practitioners who practice at separate locations and do not consult among themselves about clients.

Group Practice

The trend toward group practice stems from certain advantages, some inherent and some the result of changes in health care systems. Group practice provides a built-in mechanism for consulting with respected colleagues regularly. Many groups schedule clinical meetings to track the progress of and offer advice about clients. Groups also tend to structure themselves along a gradient of experience; for example, a typical group might consist of two senior therapists who have practiced for many years, three therapists of intermediate experience, and one recent graduate. Groups can also represent a much wider range of areas of therapeutic (and marketing!) expertise than a single individual can.

Another inherent advantage to group practice is coverage for clients in the event of illness, vacation, or professional obligation. For those of you who are concerned with the issue of "turning it off" and getting away from the 24-hour responsibility discussed on pages 11–13, the back-up support provided in a group practice may be an extremely important consideration. The lifestyle we create as independent practitioners can just as easily represent a burden, a 24-hour burden if you do not have adequate backup, as it does freedom. Therapists are different from other people in that they need to be responsible to people from the minute they say "Hello" until they say "Goodbye." Your decision to involve yourself with a group is related to the amount of time and energy you are willing to put into your practice.

A group will also be more able (financially) to hire administrative and clerical personnel to handle the business and financial record-keeping, billing and collections, and general office tasks that are necessary but that do not directly generate income. As an independent practitioner, you need to spend your time doing what you do best. What do you do best? Obviously, the therapy, but also the practice-building. Who else can build *your particular practice* better than you can? Thus, a general rule for independent practitioners is to be efficient by delegating tasks in which you are not expert. (We will talk more about this idea in the section on consultants, pp. 149–151.) If you are sharing the expenses for support staff and if you use the time you would have spent doing clerical jobs *to build your business*, your portion of the expenses will not only be efficiently used, but the compensation to you will be immense.

Being part of a group is also useful in networking. We have found that being part of a group helps those who have difficulty talking about themselves and what they do. By talking about others in your group—their areas of specialization, credentials, new things you are doing as a group or the newest member, or whatever—you infer your own competence and effectiveness. You also increase your chances of getting a referral somewhere along the line. For example, suppose you are a marriage and family therapist with a secondary specialization in chemical addiction. Jane, the person to whom you are talking at a benefit dinner, has no need of your services nor does she know anyone who does; if you were only talking about yourself that would be the end of it. You have talked about the various other therapists in your group, however; later, Jane talks about your group and passes along the name of your colleague who specializes in biofeedback to Steve, a friend of hers who has chronic pain that cannot be physically alleviated. Steve begins treatment with your colleague. Steve's coworker John (whom Jane does not know) has confided in Steve that he is worried about his son, whom he suspects may be using drugs, and the strain his son's behavior is putting on his marriage. Steve knows of just the person John and his family should see—you!

The most obvious advantage that group practice provides in the face of changes in health care is the management of liability. Management of liability does not necessarily mean reduction in your vulnerability to malpractice suits. On the one hand, groups may be more vulnerable to cavalier lawsuits because of the "deeper pockets" of a group (assuming for the moment that the group has some sort of joint liability). On the other hand, group practice may mitigate against justifiable lawsuits because misdiagnosis or inappropriate treatment is less likely. Management of liability would encompass knowledge of liability risks, clear and considered policies, and a mandate that each member be accountable to the group for adherence to those policies.

Another issue associated with the changing nature of health care delivery is that of referral sources, specifically where they will come from in the future. Personal reputation and local networks will still form the foundation from which referrals will come. However, with the growth of regional and national networks and "mega-contract" affiliations, we think an increasing percentage of referrals will result from these sources. Being associated with a group is an obvious advantage—probably a necessity in fact—to obtaining large contracts. Our feeling is that people who are well established in solo practice and/or who are in popular specialties will continue to succeed in solo practice; for new people coming into the field, joining a group practice may make more and more sense in the 1990s.

There can be some disadvantages in group practice, depending on the type of group. One difficulty normally associated with groups—lack of decision-making control—is not inevitable. The way a group practice is legally and organizationally structured determines the level of control an individual has. If the group consists of solo practitioners sharing overhead and/or clerical support, individual autonomy is comparable to the independent practitioner's. Other problems that are associated with group practice include the possibility of guilt by association. We know of, for example, an alcohol rehabilitation counselor, director of a group practice, who was arrested and convicted on several *driving under the influence* (DUI) charges; the group lost clients and eventually disbanded because the reputation of the group suffered significantly from one individual's behavior. Individual therapists can lose clients if the group disbands. Groups are also susceptible to all of the difficulties inherent in the group process including jealousies, personality conflicts, gossip, scapegoating, and power conflicts.

Solo Practice

The major advantage to solo practice is independence. The therapist determines how many hours and when he or she will work, the number and type of clients, and the extent and type of practice-building activities. Of course, the therapist is solely responsible for all clinical decisions; for some, this is the profound advantage of individual practice. With total independence, however, comes a concomitant responsibility.

For those solo practitioners who practice from their homes, low overhead is also an advantage. For new graduates and transitioning professionals, the home office is frequently perceived as ideal: no additional rent or utilities payments; availability to one's family; no commuting; lower clothing and food budget; flexibility of schedule; and freedom to engage in other activities at will (recreational, domestic, etc.). But we find this option fraught with difficulties. Experience has taught many home practitioners that the elements they perceived as advantages in fact deter the success of their practices. For example, access to family means access to disruption. Availability to alternate activities means availability to distraction. Savings in rent, food, and clothing costs can result in a lessened image of professionalism, at least in the minds of some potential clients and referral sources. Some clients may find it charming to have to step over the kitty litter to get to where they are going; others will say, "Oh, no!"

Some practitioners believe that client involvement in the therapist's personal surroundings disrupts the formation of transference. If other family members are present in a nearby space, the possibility of client restraint in expression of affect is also problematic. Another potential problem centers on lifestyle. Certain therapists practice in one lifestyle and live in another; in the home-based setting, you are opening yourself up to questions, the answers to which you may not want everybody to know. Where you live, how much you spend on your mortgage, or how big or small your house is, really is not anyone's business but yours; but if you are practicing at home, you are revealing this information whether you want to or not.

Finally, although the risks of personal assault to the practitioner and allegations by the client of impropriety on the part of the therapist are higher for the solo practitioner than for the group practitioner, they are especially salient for the home-based practice. In a home-based setting, when you are dealing with people who are homicidal or suicidal, you are putting yourself and the rest of your family at risk, and there is no way to get around it.

We are not trying to sound discouraging about the home-based practice. For some people, a home-based practice is absolutely what they want, and we say "fine." We are also saying, however, that the decision cannot simply be based on economic considerations: you have to weigh carefully factors such as who your clientele is, whom you are attracting, and the image you are putting forth.

Another option that Ralph has encountered to keep overhead low—especially directed to those fresh from school—is using a referral source's office to see clients, for example a physician's. Although this arrangement may work on a very short-term basis in individual cases, we believe the overall detriments are greater than the benefits. Again, the general issue of image needs to be considered. What image are you creating in your client *and in your referral source* by not having your own office? A lack of commitment to independent practice? An air of fly-by-night, the client or physician suspects, that may affect your competence as a therapist? If you were the physician, how inclined would you be to refer to someone who displaced you from your office—or at least moved your piles of paper and your coffee cup—every time he or she saw a client?

One arrangement that may work, however, is to sublet space from a physician/group of physicians. In this situation, you might be positioning yourself very well for referrals and clerical/administrative support while keeping your overhead fairly low. Identity issues might still be problematic, though, resulting in a lack of referrals beyond the physician(s); privacy might also be a problem. When Ralph began his independent practice (after he had lived in Phoenix long enough to make substantial community contacts), he was associated with a group of OB/GYN physicians. The group helped him get going and generally known in town as a solo practitioner, as well as recognized in the medical community as a family therapist. On the negative side, however, he became known as a person with that particular group; that is, other physicians were afraid to refer to him for fear the physicians with whom he was associated would steal the outside referring physicians' clients.

Executive suites offer another possibility for the solo practitioner. These range from a single office to a cluster of offices. Often the buildings offer a package of services from which you can select: clerical, reception, telephone, and computer. Rent is based on size and location of the office, term of the lease, and services chosen. This structure can enhance the appearance of professionalism at a moderate cost. Of course, the traditional choice of the solo practitioner is the self-sustaining arrangement—practitioner, perhaps support staff, in an office(s) within a building occupied by other tenants or occupying its own building. (See Chapter 7 for a more complete discussion of the therapist's office.)

BUSINESS STRUCTURE

In legal terms, there are three types of business organization—sole proprietorship, partnership, and corporation—with advantages and disadvantages to each, depending on the type of practice and market you have chosen. As we advise in Chapter 8, we are not in the business of giving legal advice. The decision about what business structure is best suited to your needs should only be made in consultation with your tax accountant and an attorney.

Sole Proprietorship

If you are in a solo practice, you will probably have a sole proprietorship. This is the simplest, least expensive business arrangement. No organizational documentation is required, and you have absolute authority over all decisions. A sole proprietorship is not taxed as a business entity; business income is taxed as personal income, and losses/expenses are deductible (Minars, 1987). (Depending on your total income, this taxation procedure can be an advantage or disadvantage.) Upon your death or retirement, there is no formal mechanism required to transfer or sell the practice. What you must remember, however, is that often you must obtain certain types of business operating licenses. Almost every jurisdiction has some kind of occupational license. You do not need a lawyer to get a license, though you may want to consult with one to find out what licenses are required. The procedure is simple, but failure to obtain a business license could leave you open to a malpractice suit. You must also check zoning requirements, especially if you are practicing or plan to practice in your home. Frequently, a zoning check is part of the business license procedure but not necessarily.

The major disadvantage of a sole proprietorship is that it subjects you to unlimited personal liability; if you are sued and the judgment is against you, all of your assets—home, car, personal possessions—may be used in the settlement. This personal liability is of two types: professional, in which you are liable for malpractice if you allegedly err in your practice, and the more general liability of being responsible if someone walks into your office, falls, and breaks a leg. (See Chapter 8 for a discussion of professional liability; general liability is discussed in Chapter 7 under the heading of insurance, pp. 151–155.) The other main disadvantage of a sole proprietorship is that all profits automatically accrue to the owner, which may put the individual in a very high tax bracket (Minars, 1987).

Partnership

In a partnership, two or more people agree to share ownership, profits, and sometimes management of a business. Partners can be general or limited. General partners participate in the day-to-day operations of the business and are personally liable for the business's obligations. Limited partners do not participate in management responsibilities or authority and are liable only to the extent of their investment. A partnership must have at least one general partner. Limited partners are usually brought in to provide more capital for the business. For example, you might form a limited partnership with a parent or spouse who agrees to pay the first six months' rent on your office in return for a percentage of the profits. As in the sole proprietorship, income in a partnership is taxed as personal income and losses/expenses are tax deductible.

Partnerships seem to be an area of confusion for therapists. Some form of sharing revenue is the classic test for a partnership, though the sharing does not have to be equal. In the experience of Steven L. Engelberg, a partner in Keck, Mahin, and Cate, which serves as legal counsel to the American Association for Marriage and Family Therapists (AAMFT), some therapists may be operating in a relationship that resembles a partnership but is not (Law and Ethics Workshop, April 20, 1987, Tucson, Arizona). Many therapists identify themselves as partners in group practice, but these groups are often more cost-sharing arrangements rather than partnerships pooling their revenues. Although you do not intend to be a partnership, if you are not careful, there are circumstances in which the law may impose a partnership and its concurrent liability on you. Most states define how a partnership should operate in their jurisdiction. For example, you have an office-sharing arrangement with three other therapist-tenants. You are each operating independently, but you share the costs of a secretary, office equipment, and general overhead. You even give yourselves a name, which is technically allowed but can easily, if you are not careful, lead clients, vendors, and so on to believe you are a partnership. In certain cases, state law will in effect impose a partnership on you.

Why should you be concerned if the law considers your arrangement a partnership, even if you and your office mates have not drawn up a partnership agreement and do not intend to operate as a partnership? In a partnership, each person is the agent of the other partners; what this means is that **you are responsible, liable, for the others' actions.** If one person in this arrangement is sued, the others can be named as partners in the lawsuit. If you have chosen to enter into a formal partnership, then you recognize this joint liability up front. You are partners for purposes of professional liability as well as for profits and other commercial purposes. Suppose one general partner orders a $10,000 computer without consulting the others. The others may think the idea a bad one and refuse to pay for the purchase. But too bad—all general partners are personally liable for each other's actions. Unlike a corporation, a partnership is not a separate, taxable entity. If a partnership is sued or goes bankrupt, the assets are the personal assets of the partners. The partner with more personal assets will probably lose more.

The key factor is how you hold yourself up to the public at large. You cannot present the public with the image that you are a group, and all for one and everybody is together, if you are not; otherwise, you run the risk of the state imposing its definition of a partnership on you. In other words, you cannot have your cake and eat it too. If you do not want to run the risk of looking like a partnership, you must make it clear that you are all separate practitioners, even if you operate from a suite of offices with a common reception area. For example, you each put your name outside the main door and individually on your separate offices. You do not hand out literature that suggests you are in business with the other people, and appointments are made separately. If a client calls one of the other therapists, he or she does not get you.

What if you want to draw up a formal partnership agreement? You should consult a lawyer, *who is familiar with partnership law in the state in which you practice*, to draw up an agreement spelling out the specifics of the arrangement. (In some states, you *must* draw up such an agreement to avoid violating state law.) There are certain issues that must be addressed or you may invoke the default provisions of state-determined partnerships laws. These issues will vary by state. One area you will probably need to define is decision-making. You can have a partnership with one dominant partner if you so desire, or you can decide to have a one-person, one-vote arrangement. If you do not spell this out in the agreement, however, the state may declare, for example, that the decision-making is by majority vote. Similarly, state law may declare that partnership profits are to be shared equally. Again, other arrangements may be perfectly acceptable, but they must be spelled out in writing. (There are such things as oral partnerships, but they are sometimes very difficult to enforce.)

Another issue that may need to be dealt with in a formal partnership is continuity. In many states, the death or withdrawal of one partner automatically dissolves the entire partnership. If you are partners with more than one person, you obviously do not want this to happen, so again you must specify in writing what will happen in the event of death or withdrawal of one partner.

Of course the main issue involved in a partnership is one we have already mentioned—the issue of liability. Each partner is your agent and can literally bind you and the partnership to whatever act he or she carries out, including alleged professional malpractice. Traditionally, therapists who prescribe medications, that is, psychiatrists, have been sued more frequently and for greater amounts than those who practice the so-called "talking therapies." While large judgments against non-psychiatrists are not that common, lawsuits are becoming more prevalent every day. Thus, the fact that you can be sued for someone else's act may be more important because of the threat of lawsuits in the first place, and not necessarily because of ultimate judgments and amounts (Law and Ethics Workshop, April 20, 1987).

Deciding whether or not the benefits of a partnership outweigh the potential problems with liability is an individual decision. We emphatically recommend that you engage a lawyer to draw up a partnership agreement if you do decide to form a partnership. He or she can advise you about what issues should be covered and various alternatives to standard arrangements that can be tailored to your particular practice. Your professional life is too important to play amateur lawyer. One of the points we have repeated throughout this book is to do what you do best and build a team for yourself that includes the services of others doing what they do best.

Incorporation

One of the primary reasons for incorporating is to shield yourself from liability. Unlike sole proprietorships and partnerships, corporations are autonomous legal entities. Ownership of a corporation is freely transferable, and a corporation does not cease to exist if the owner or partners die. Most salient, perhaps, is the provision that the liability of all shareholders is limited to the amount they have invested. The bad news, however, is that there is a fundamental difference between a professional business and a nonprofessional business: Professionals cannot shield themselves from professional liability (malpractice) by incorporating. Many states have specific laws that allow professionals to incorporate and spell out ways incorporation should be handled. Other states do not have such laws.

In neither case, however, are you necessarily protected from the threat of suit. For example, suppose you are in solo practice but want to set yourself up as a corporation. (State regulations vary on whether or not this is allowed.) Assuming for the moment your state does allow this, you file the proper legal documents and add "Inc." to the name of your practice. A client decides to sue you for alleged inappropriate diagnosis and treatment. You probably cannot respond by saying, "Wait, I'm off the hook. I'm not individually liable because I'm incorporated." In Engelberg's opinion, the court is more likely to say, "Tough. You are an individual professional performing services. You can't hide behind a corporate shield" (Law and Ethics Workshop, April 20, 1987). This is a very different situation from a plumber coming into your house, running amuck, and being as negligent as possible. If the plumber is properly incorporated and properly maintaining a corporation, you probably cannot sue the plumber but must go after the corporation.

If you are a solo practitioner, reasons to incorporate will most likely focus on certain tax considerations. To figure out your individual situation, we advise you to consult with a good accountant. Many of the traditional tax advantages for corporations have fallen by the wayside as a result of changes in tax law. For example, some years ago when Engelberg set up his law firm as a professional corporation, the firm could set up a retirement plan and defer much more money than it could if it had been a sole proprietorship or partnership. Since that time, the law has been changed so that this discrepancy no longer exists (Law and Ethics Workshop, April 20, 1987). The 1986 Tax Reform Law with its uniform 28 percent taxation rate also mitigates against many previous corporate tax advantages. Subsequent tax reform activity may or may not alter your particular situation.

Sub-Chapter S

An intermediate structure between a corporation and a partnership is the "Sub-Chapter S" corporation. Sub-S corporations are small corporations with fewer than 35 stockholders (Minars, 1987). In this structure, the corporation is taxed like a partnership, that is, the corporation's incomes or losses are credited or debited to the stockholders in proportion to their holdings, and there is no taxation at the corporate level. The S-corporation will also protect you against personal (non-professional) liability and may offer some tax advantages regarding long-term capital gains (Minars, 1987). The value of this structure for your business is best decided by you and your attorney.

In Engelberg's opinion, if you are in solo practice, whether or not you incorporate is probably not a "life or death" situation though he cautions that each person should make this decision only in consultation with his or her lawyer (Law and Ethics Workshop, April 20, 1987). If you are practicing as a group and you intend to operate like a partnership, you may want to consider forming a corporation, because there are certain ways of incorporating that will facilitate decision making, continuity, and other issues discussed in the section on partnerships. Also, be aware that in certain states, if you plan to incorporate a group, you are going to have difficulty combining some professions in this corporation. In some states, a psychologist can only form a partnership with another licensed psychologist. In other states multidisciplinary corporations are legal. We reiterate: as a practicing professional, decisions about whether or not you *can* incorporate and whether or not you *should* incorporate require sensitive legal judgment; unless you can afford to be cavalier in your decision, we recommend you consult a business attorney for advice.

7/
From Design to Detail: Office Planning, Policies, and Procedures

THE THERAPIST'S OFFICE

Your office is a statement of your marketing and therapeutic image. The location, design, and furniture will communicate to those who visit definite ideas about your approach to the practice of therapy and business. For example, the Gestalt therapist's office will frequently have props, pillows, additional chairs, and space for moving about. The more traditional office might be furnished with a desk with a chair on either side. A three-inch plush carpet might suggest how you are spending the $85 per hour fee. You need to assess the impact of these statements on your particular market. What might be expected or reassuring to some clients may be threatening or annoying to others.

One idea we believe is a myth—or a mistake—is the notion of "well, I'd like to have an office that fits in with a certain level of clientele (those who can afford to pay), but I'm just starting out and can't swing the overhead, so I'll start with low overhead (for example, office in the home or in a certain geographic location, secondhand/inadequate furniture) and change to a higher overhead (a more distinctive office) when my practice is established." The problem with this idea is that changing the image established by your first office may be tougher and take longer than you think. If you try to cut overhead too much when you are beginning and project a certain image, through subsequent referrals and feedback, that image may follow you in the community for a long time.

Location

Location is the first consideration for your office's image. Common sense tells us to consider such locational aspects as adequate parking, convenience to the target market, easy access to main thoroughfares and bus lines, ambiance of the neighborhood, and zoning regulations. A demographic study might be useful. Ralph's facility, for example, is located in Scottsdale one block away from Scottsdale Hospital, one of the main general hospitals in Scottsdale, and a block and a half from Camelback Hospital, the largest psychiatric hospital system in the metropolitan Phoenix area. The area serves as a hub for the entire valley, and referrals come from Phoenix, Tempe, Scottsdale, Chandler, Gilbert, Glendale—in all, about 1.8 million people are encompassed by this area. Marketing research has shown that more people in the area, for various reasons, will go into Scottsdale for professional services.

In addition to these fairly obvious considerations, you need to consider the issue of client privacy. When Joan's group decided to open their office, they first looked at offices in a very large bank building. The group realized they did not want to be located where clients such as doctors and lawyers would bump into their accountants or people with whom they meet in their own offices. The group finally decided upon a remodeled convenience store in a centrally located, well-established, residential neighborhood. The setting is quiet, relaxed, and most of all private; even the parking lot is surrounded by a seven-foot hedge of oleanders. People will say to Joan, "It doesn't look like a convenience store. It looks like a first-class building." She will often respond, "Currently I work in the slurpee section, and someday I may work in dairy products." When making a decision about an office located with other offices, the therapist needs to ask himself or herself, "Who are my neighbors? How much risk is there of my clients running into my neighbors? How will my clients feel if they do?''

Layout

The layout of your office(s) is also important for therapeutic reasons. There is no single correct floor plan for an office. You should, however, keep some basic principles in mind. First, for certain clients a separate entrance and exit is important. Many people—especially those who are prominent in the community—do not want to be seen by others leaving a therapist's office. Some people are sensitive about being seen by other clients if they have had an especially emotional session. We have always stressed a wellness model of therapy—both for therapeutic and business reasons. But until this model is accepted by a substantial public majority, the therapist must be sensitive to people's (real or imagined) fears about the stigma attached to therapy. On the other hand, many clients also seem to enjoy talking to other clients. In Joan's experience, clients frequently discuss therapy or other topics in her group practice's common waiting room. (In these circumstances it is very important to try not to schedule two people from the same organization at the same time.) Another privacy issue pertains to sound-proofing. Make sure your office is constructed well enough or located far enough away so that clients who are waiting and your support staff cannot hear the therapy sessions taking place in your office.

Furnishings

In thinking about furnishings for your office—though this idea also pertains to location and layout—keep in mind that the space in which you practice must be a background, and not an interruption, to the therapeutic process. It may be helpful to think of furnishing your office in a way that somehow reflects the lifestyle of your clients and fits into the neighborhood environment surrounding your office. You convey messages both of who you are and who your clients are with art, color, furniture style, and plants; even the magazines in your waiting room convey images of you and your clients.

Both of us believe in creating a flexible, comfortable, living room setting; that is our bias based on our identities as marriage and family therapists. As we mentioned in Chapter 3, however, context is everything—hot tubs would be a bit too relaxed and casual for our particular clientele, as would 40-year-old, overstuffed chairs with the stuffing coming out from Aunt Mathilde's attic. And you do not want to charge $60, $70, or $100 an hour and make your clients sit on stools and folding chairs. At the same time, creating an office that looks like something from a penthouse suite in New York (unless you happen to practice among the very well-to-do in New York) may also be a poor choice. You do not want your clients to resent your fee because they think it is all going into plush carpeting and collectors' items.

Support Services and Support Staff

Support services in your office are critical, especially surrounding the telephone. Even if you are on a tight budget and are looking for the lowest possible overhead, we believe an answering service AND NOT AN ANSWERING MACHINE is preferable. You do not want to come back to a machine and hear your client say, "I took 142 pills at 3:42 on Friday afternoon and goodbye," and it is now Wednesday and a lawyer wants to know what kind of coverage you have and who is responsible. In addition, many people get anxious or angry about having to talk to a machine; they want to talk to a human being, especially if they are distressed. Not all answering services are alike, however, and a poor one is almost as bad as having none at all. Before you sign up with any service, ask these questions:

1. Who are your customers? Are any of them therapists?
2. Will you provide 24-hour coverage?

3. Will the same people handle my calls or will they be answered randomly? What is the average length of employment of your employees?
4. May I select the people who handle my calls and train them?
5. Does your staff handle emergency situations for other clients?
6. What is the protocol for calling me? How quickly will I be called?
7 May I script your staff's responses to my calls and rehearse them?
8. How are fees determined—flat fee, per call, or another way?

If these questions seem overly detailed or picky, remember that the person answering your telephone creates the first impression of your business (meaning, you) in the minds of clients, potential clients, and referral sources. You may be the best therapist in the world, but if your initial contact via the telephone with the public is unpleasant, less than professional, or incompetent, you will never have the opportunity to practice that therapy on any client. Once you have selected a service and you visit the facility to sign the contract, we suggest that you humanize the relationship. For example, bring the answering service staff cookies or fruit or flowers; learn their names. You may want to make periodic visits to the service because of employee turnover. You may also want to arrange for a friend or colleague to call your service occasionally and offer you feedback. You want the service personnel to realize you are serious and professional about what you do. In turn, they will treat your clients with respect and dignity and extend your professional image. When we are treating people with real dilemmas, we need support staff who will perceive emergencies as genuine.

We recognize that not all therapists will be able to find an acceptable answering service and will choose to use an answering machine. If you do, your message should reflect your professionalism and concern. Clients find it helpful when the message contains information about when you will be available and how often you check your machine. You may also want to include an emergency number where you, a colleague, or hospital emergency staff (with whom you have a coverage arrangement) can be reached. Here is a sample message:

Hello. This is Connie Smith. Please leave your name, number, the time you called, and any message after the beep. I will be calling in for messages this evening at 7 and 10. You can reach me at this number tomorrow morning after 8. If you have an emergency, please call my colleague Sally Jones (or Community Hospital) at 123-1234. Thank you.

You will want to purchase an answering machine that is voice-activated (allowing any length of message) and enables you to check-in from any phone. The most convenient type of remote access does not require a hand-held device but rather is activated with a numerical code.

More therapists are choosing to carry beepers, at least part of the time. In group practices, therapists take turns being on call. Using a beeper can be a cost-effective alternative to an answering service and is far better than spending your time on call within earshot of your telephone.

If you are in a practice that can support a receptionist and/or secretary, the same principles apply. It is your responsibility to make sure your staff not only represents you in a friendly, concerned, and professional manner, but also that they are trained to truly *support* your efficacy as a practitioner. This is particularly true when they are called on to recognize and react to emergencies. A staff member in Joan's practice exemplified this principle when she answered a call from a client trying to reach Joan. The client was very distressed but vague about her crisis level. Joan was temporarily unavailable. Rather than just referring the call to the on-call therapist, the staff member choose to contact the client's neighbor who was a therapist in Joan's group (and had referred the client to Joan). The staff member called the neighbor/therapist and shared her concerns about the client. The neighbor arrived at the client's home and discovered the client had swallowed a vial of barbiturates just minutes before. The staff member's compassion and willingness to act saved the client's life.

We are biased in favor of having at least one full-time support person if you are in full-time independent practice. A secretary, office manager, or receptionist can tie many threads together. He or she can be the original contact person both on the phone and in person, thus creating a comfortable sense of continuity for the client. Handling the phones is especially important when you are in session. We know some therapists who take all calls themselves, even while they are in session. Some are able to do this tactfully. We do not believe this is in clients' best interests because it disrupts the special relationship therapy represents. In addition, a secretary or bookkeeper can be responsible for making contractual billing and payment arrangements with clients, freeing the therapist from that role. We believe support staff more than pay for themselves, in that the therapist gains additional time to take on more clients and engage in activities to market the business—activities that actually result in payback—rather than spending his or her time in nonpaid administrative tasks.

If you are in independent practice part-time, obviously a full-time support person may not make much sense. We urge you, however, to consider hiring a support person in conjunction with other therapists or other professionals. For instance, you could arrange with two other colleagues in part-time independent practice—not necessarily in the same location, though proximity would be useful—to divide the services of one full-time person. Perhaps you would have the secretary for fifteen hours a week, your colleague for another fifteen hours, and the third colleague for ten. Employee benefits and required contributions such as FICA, unemployment insurance, and worker's compensation can be split along percentages tied in to the proportion of hours. We caution you, however, to consult with your attorney about this arrangement if there is any question of implied partnership (see Chapter 6, pp. 118-121).

Even though we urge hiring support staff, we recognize that many successful practices are one-person operations. For example, William Nichols built his practice without the aid of a staff. In fact, he went so far as to use an answering machine rather than a service because he was dissatisfied with the service's performance. He says, "It's possible—if you can type billing statements fairly well and an occasional insurance form or report—to gross $100,000 or so without supporting other people in your office. Also, if you don't use support staff, you don't have to gross as much because you don't have to carry them" (Personal Communication, October 1988).

You as an Employer

Of course, hiring employees places you in the role of employer. The most important element of your role as an employer is the establishment of your personnel policies. Bonnie McKnight, regional manager of Payroll Tax Control Corporation in Los Angeles, consults in the areas of human resources and payroll tax cost-containment procedures (see sections on Unemployment Insurance (pp. 157-159) and Worker's Compensation (pp. 159-160) in this chapter). She notes that therapists are particularly suited to and challenged by their attempts to develop personnel policies and practices (Personal Communication, April 1989). Therapeutic communication skills can be effective in hiring, retaining, and developing personnel. However, even the best therapist can find it difficult to separate the role of therapist from that of employer, both of which involve similar power dynamics. To keep the employer-employee relationship clear, McKnight recommends that the employer establish and administer well thought-out policies and procedures (Personal Communication, April 1988). This process requires that

1. The employer develop standardized personnel policies and practices;
2. Each employee receive a written copy of the personnel policies and practices, which should include a signature page that indicates the employee has read and understood the contents;
3. The employer take care to apply all practices consistently and fairly.

McKnight further suggests practices that will tend to limit employee dissatisfaction and therefore turnover (McKnight, 1988). Particularly for the independent practitioner, employee turnover can be quite troublesome. Clients often learn to trust your staff, and their observations are at times useful clinically. To support job satisfaction, McKnight recommends that you implement the following general suggestions:

1. Regardless of the job function, ensure that all employees understand the relation of their jobs to other jobs within the practice and that they see how their jobs contribute to the final outcome;
2. Educate the employees on the role of your services, how therapy is of benefit to clients;
3. Make employees fully aware of their job responsibilities and what is expected of them, endeavoring to avoid the "that's not part of my job" attitude;
4. Do not make promises or commitments that cannot be kept;
5. Provide thorough, meaningful performance appraisals to ensure that the employees know where they stand. Acknowledge strengths, achievements, and areas needing improvement, offer specific suggestions on how to improve;
6. Establish some type of suggestion system. When appropriate, ask employees for ideas and always respond to their input;
7. The greater the number of ways you have for employees to voice their concerns about their work and their working conditions, the lower your turnover will be. Make it easy for employees to speak up—then show employees you listen by responding appropriately;
8. Keep employees apprised of relevant policy changes and other miscellaneous practice matters that affect them; and
9. Supervision and management need to project a positive attitude toward the practice and the employees; negativity breeds negativity. (McKnight, 1988, reprinted with permission)

Computers in the Therapist's Office

As they are in many walks of life, computers are fast becoming an everyday part of the therapist's practice. There are two main types of computer applications for the therapist's office: clerical and clinical.

Clerical applications handle such functions as word processing, billing, accounting, scheduling and administrative reporting. According to Jeff Stull, who is a partner in Desert Data, a software development firm in Scottsdale, the majority of the software packages developed specifically for the therapist's clerical tasks have focused on insurance and billing procedures because these areas are so much more complicated for the therapist than, for example, the physician (Personal Communication, December 1989). A few packages, such as Desert Data's, integrate scheduling, billing, and accounting functions. Stull points to a number of advantages good software can provide (Personal Communication, December 1989):

1. *Savings in Staff Costs.* With a computer to handle a number of clerical functions, fewer staff members are required to run an office. In addition, entering data into a computer requires much less skill than doing the accounting or record-keeping manually.

2. *Consistency.* Computer software forces you to standardize your records and methods. If the software is properly matched to your office procedures, the computer can save you and your support staff time and effort. Establishing consistency in record-keeping, billing, and accounting, and so on, is especially important in a group practice, where each individual may come to the group with his or her own way of handling these tasks.

3. *Professionalism.* Manual procedures may be appropriate for a very small or very new practice, but as a practice grows, patients tend to expect more emphasis on efficiency and up-to-date information professionally packaged and presented.

4. *Business Planning.* Computers can generate sophisticated analyses of profits and losses, referral activity,

reimbursement trends, and so on. These analyses can be invaluable in developing marketing plans.

Therapists routinely cite lack of time, lack of training, or the size of their practice (too small to justify the expense) as reasons for not using computers (Farrell, 1989). Therapists also express some concern about the appropriateness of computer use in their offices, especially for clinical tasks. Although more and more therapists are using computers for clerical functions, there seems to be much more resistance to using them for clinical functions, with the exception of test-scoring (Farrell, 1989). These clinical applications include such tasks as assigning diagnoses, gathering client data, conducting biofeedback, and conducting cognitive retraining. Most therapists still seem to prefer employing other professionals for these tasks.

It is clear that the development of both clerical and clinical applications is burgeoning but still very young. While general computer literacy is rising, access to information about specialized applications for the mental health professional is limited (Farrell, 1989). Stull recommends talking to colleagues with experience in computer use and attending professional meetings to gather information about software packages. He also points out that more professional journals and magazines are beginning to include software reviews (Personal Communication, December 1989). Farrell (1989) believes that more continuing education classes that improve therapists' knowledge and train them in the appropriate use of computers in their practice need to be offered.

FEES, PAYMENT, BILLING, AND COLLECTIONS

It is hard to say whether "marketing" or "money" is the more dreaded "M-word." In any case, the two are so intertwined that much of what we said in the early chapters of this book should probably be repeated at this point. Instead, we will simply assume that if you need to, you will go back and re-read material having to do with "permission" to make money, unrealistic dichotomizing between the helper and entrepreneur, and so on. The basic issue about money, about being paid for the product of therapy, is "How much do I value what I do?" Although the following statement may sound glib or oversimplified, there is some fundamental truth to it. If the answer to the question is that you truly value what you do, then money issues will cease to be quite so problematic once you have done some planning and have made decisions about procedures. If, however, the answer to the question is that you do not value what you do (enough to ask for and expect a fair return on your labor), then you should perhaps ask yourself why you are in this line of work.

Steven Engelberg, the attorney whom we quoted in Chapter 6, offers an interesting perspective on the issue of money (fees, billing, collections) and its relationship to the helping side of our profession. He says, speaking of his profession and of ours,

I believe we have a duty to do more than make money; we also have a duty to give something back. We all have a duty to do pro bono work, but one reason we often don't prefer to do pro bono work is that we are wasting our time with a lot of deadbeats who can afford to pay and don't pay, people who won't deal with us in a commercially fair way. In your commercial time, make sure you are commercial. Don't lose what you have earned (from those who can afford to pay) to unreasonably low fee-setting or sloppy billing and collection. (I call the latter "legal enrichment services," because I have seen therapists repeatedly paying for legal services and spending time they could be devoting to pro bono work, trying to collect in situations that are the fault of unclear expectations or their actual billing and/or collection procedures.) (Law and Ethics Workshop, April 20, 1987, Tucson, Ariz.)

The therapist has an ethical duty to be very clear about what is expected of the client concerning the entire financial procedure—from clearly delineated fees to the billing, payment, and collection arrangements. Certainly this is important as a protection against litigation. Many therapists also believe it is important to the therapeutic process. The therapist, after clearly spelling out the terms—how much and when—must then *expect* that the client will fulfill his or her part of the contract and also make that expectation clear to the client. Finally the therapist must *follow up* with the client along the lines of the original agreement. (See Appendix II for sample agreement forms.)

Setting Fees

There is nothing hard and fast about the first part of the process, setting fees. You need to gather as much data as you can about fee structures. Publications such as *Psychotherapy Finances* periodically give national fee structures and averages. Data on particular types of therapists (psychiatrists, psychologists, marriage and family therapists, for example) are usually available from professional organizations. You should also contact local colleagues in your area of specialization because particular geographic areas may differ widely from the average. For example, a city with a disproportionately high number of marriage and family therapists may only support a lower than average fee; this situation may be modified, however, for a particular therapist if she or he has a subspecialty not well represented in this city. Finally, you should contact third-party payers to find out what their maximum allowance is. Keep in mind, though, that you may want to set your fees higher than third-party payers currently allow because fee scales for a given year are frequently based on the median from the previous year (Ridgewood Financial Institute, 1984).

If you want to raise your fees, the same kind of homework is useful. Some therapists raise their fees only for new clients, keeping current clients at the fee at which they began. This can create record-keeping and billing nightmares and increase the chances that you will bill some clients in error, all of which can contribute to collection problems. We find it preferable to begin telling all of your current clients, at least three months in advance, that you will be raising your fees, occasionally repeating this information in subsequent sessions. In our experience, most clients are amenable to the change if they have sufficient notice to prepare for it. As they come in, new clients are also told upfront of the impending change.

Therapists who are just beginning in the field or who are new to independent practice are often tempted to set fairly low fees. While this is an individual decision, and can sometimes bolster a practice (as, for example, if you work out an arrangement with a senior practitioner whereby he or she regularly sends you clients referred to him or her who cannot afford that practitioner's fees), in our experience, we find it preferable to set fees comparable to our colleagues' fee structures. We believe it is important to your own sense of self-worth as well as to your professional image and standing among your colleagues. A story in *Psychotherapy Finances Guide to Private Practice* told of one therapist who reported that any therapist in her area who charged less than the going rate was accused of undercutting the competition; referrals began to dry up. According to the *Guide*, "Rather than get into a hassle over the moral and legal implications of this type of price fixing, the therapist reported that she refers patients who can't pay her full fee to a local social agency where she works part-time, and then sees them for the agency's usual sliding scale" (Ridgewood Financial Institute, 1984, Section 3, p. 4).

Varying fee structures within groups can create potentially sticky situations. In Joan's group, everyone is an independent contractor and sets his or her own fees. They discuss the fees, but no one is told what to charge. Two social workers refuse to go over $50 per hour; two psychiatrists refuse to see anyone for under $100. Both of these are accepted among the group. A client may say, "Why does someone charge $50 and this other one is $85?" Joan responds with, "Both of these people have competence in what they are doing, both have been in the field a long time, and this is what they choose to charge." Neither of us chooses to use sliding fee scales, though we are certainly not telling you not to use them. In our experience, the added paperwork and the potential for misrepresentation outweigh the supposed marketing advantage. Additionally, this practice is uncommon outside the mental health field. We prefer to reduce a fee when a particular situation warrants it.

One practice that Joan has found to be an excellent marketing tool and a way to build client relations regarding fees is to not charge for intake and termination sessions. "I give them a present for good health. Nobody who is doing well and feeling good wants to come back and say, 'Joan, you were terrific' for $70. People walk out saying, 'I'll pay,' but I say, 'It's present enough for me to know you're doing well.' Then they can come back for a three-month or six-month check-up, and we terminate over a period of time." Not charging for the intake averts potential problems with people whom you want to refer elsewhere. In addition, collection for intake and termination sessions is often harder than that over the course of therapy. Joan thinks that in the long run her practice saves money by eliminating staff hours and paperwork required to collect from intake and termination sessions. The counterpart to the way Joan deals with intake fees is Ralph's method. Ralph collects the fee for the first session up front so as to avoid collection problems and possible lawsuits by people who only show up once. This problem is discussed in greater detail in the next section.

One issue that we would like to mention at this point is that of fee-splitting. Fee-splitting occurs when Practitioner A refers a client to Practitioner B and receives a portion of the client's fee. This can bear serious resemblance to fee-for-referral. At the very least it is inappropriate and is actually unethical. This practice, however, should not be confused with the practice of interoffice referral within a group practice. As in the previous situation, both practitioners may benefit financially; however, in this case the client is well aware of this fact. The distinction is one of secrecy versus obviousness.

A final caveat about setting fees: do not charge clients with insurance a different fee than those without insurance. You also should not waive copayments as a general policy. In certain cases, courts have ruled these practices insurance fraud. You always have the option to reduce the fee or waive the copayment for a particular client.

Payment Arrangements, Billing, and Collections

While we do not use sliding fee scales, we do use sliding payment arrangements. Joan uses the following method:

I say to the client, "Dennis, my fee is $70 a session. If you would like to pay that weekly that would be wonderful." If Dennis says "yes," I say "thank you" and shut my mouth. End of discussion. If Dennis says "no," I say, "The next opportunity we have is for you to pay it monthly." If Dennis says, "I would prefer that because I don't like to carry a check every time I come," then I say nothing more. However, Dennis may say, "That's a lot of money," especially because when I work with families I generally see them more frequently than once a week during the first month; then later spread it out to every 10 days or so. The amount of money involved in the first month may be exorbitant compared to what they can afford to pay. I will say to them, "Between this week and next, why don't you think about how much you can afford a month? I have no idea the first time I see you whether I am going to see you for six sessions or 12 or 40. You decide what you can pay per month." Usually the client will come in the next week and say something like, "I can afford $150 a month." And I'll say, "When do you get paid?" Dennis will say, "the fifth," and I'll say, "I expect a payment from you by the tenth of the month." We have internal financial forms that we fill out with the particular arrangement and the client signs it. We put it into the computer and he pays as arranged. There's no interest, or nonsense like that. Our new intake form asks for banks and account numbers. Some people say, "Not me. I'm not filling this out." I say, "It has nothing to do with you personally. It has to do with the fact that Tucson is a transient community and we have to have certain information. If you want to pay each time, you don't have to fill it out." Some people do pay each time and that's wonderful. Others fill out the form.

We recognize not everyone is going to be comfortable with this approach and may not be able to deal with clients in this way. There is disagreement among therapists about whether or not the business of payment/collections is part of the therapeutic process. In his practice—another advantage of a group—Ralph has a comptroller: a bookkeeper who gives clients a specific standardized contract, which they sign, that says "I agree to pay at each session." If they cannot do this, they work out a payment plan with the bookkeeper, who also does the collections, thus adding continuity to the process. From the beginning, the contract makes clear what they will pay each month.

In general, payment can take the form of cash (check), charge (VISA, Mastercard, etc.), or insurance. Although accepting charge cards represents an additional cost to us, we have found it encourages patient responsibility for payment.

Bartering

Barter is another form of payment about which therapists disagree. We think bartering raises at least two potentially thorny issues. First, by law, bartered items or services need to be declared as income for tax purposes. Some people may conveniently "forget" to do this, leaving themselves open to charges of tax fraud. In addition, an accurate estimate of value is sometimes difficult to document, and people may be tempted to deflate a value for tax purposes or have a hard time proving the value in the event of an audit. Second, a bartering arrangement may constitute a dual relationship. That is, the bartering arrangement may take unfair and unethical advantage of the client because of the therapeutic relationship. (See Chapter 8 for a discussion of legal implication of dual relationships.) For these reasons we discourage bartering.

When Joan first started out, she did some of bartering because she was scared she wouldn't have any clients if she did not:

I ended up with with more weavings than I knew what to do with. I had weavings coming out of my ears. Everybody got weavings for Channukah and Christmas that year. I don't do that now. Over time, I stopped bartering because of the ethical issues involved.

Bartering *can* be empowering for clients in terms of their feeling good about being able to give you something of themselves (more than money). Joan has bartered occasionally with local artists with positive results. The process must always respect therapeutic boundaries.

There can be other problems with bartering. For example, if you are doing couples work, it is very important that if you barter with one partner, the other partner does not see the situation as your getting close to the bartering partner. The times you barter should be out of the house and out of everyday vistas. You should make sure you really want and/or need what is being offered. Setting a price can be tricky, too. You should ask the person what he or she would charge if the product or service were offered in a store or business. Written documentation of the value is important. Accounting considerations can get, in Ralph's terms, "sticky"; he too did some bartering during his first year of practice, but has since given it up. Ralph further shares the concern of many other therapists who believe that bartering can interfere with the transference process. In the end, we have to say we do not encourage bartering because of the ethical issues involved. Further, on this point we think it is important to follow the ethics code of whatever professional organization(s) to which you belong.

Cancellations and No-Shows

As in any service business, cancellations and no-shows can disrupt anticipated cash flow. The therapist needs to establish a clear payment policy for missed appointments. In Ralph's practice, if people do not cancel 24 hours in advance, they are charged a full fee. Some therapists charge half-fees and some do not charge. Ralph states,

I want, as that person's therapist (and it's never the secretary who makes the decision), to make the decision to not charge if the client has a good reason for not showing up. We have a "super bill" we send to the insurance companies (see the next section on Third-party Payment), and we put "no-show" on it. It's interesting that we have seldom had a problem with the insurance company for a situation where we charge for a session and the patient didn't come. We talked to some insurance carriers about it. We put down the fee and "no-show," sometimes they pay for it and sometimes they don't. But we never go after the insurance companies for payment. If we have a collection problem with a client, we delete the "no-show" sessions. I don't want to end up with a collection agency or in Small Claims Court because of those sessions. The other side is that we get 75 to 80 percent of the claims paid anyway—full fee. Our clients understand that if they don't call to cancel ahead of time, other professionals besides therapists will charge for their time.

Joan handles "no-shows" somewhat differently.

If someone doesn't show the first time, I'll wait until two or three hours later and call and say, "I wondered what was happening. We had an appointment this morning." (In my youth, I used to call about ten minutes after the time the client was supposed to be there, and the client would come racing down and want a full session, and I decided I could use my time more productively.) If the client comes up with something plausible—"The car broke." "My son got sick."— generally I will not charge. I pay attention to it, though, and write "no-show because . . ." in my date book. I don't know how many of you know the story about how if one person tells you that you look like a horse, you can ignore him or her; if three or four people tell you that you look like a horse, you think about it but then decide they are crazy; if 18 people tell you that you look like a horse, you'd better go out and buy a saddle. There are many reasons for behaviors. If a client frequently misses appointments, obviously the action becomes a therapeutic issue. If many of your clients miss many appointments, the issue may be yours.

Collections

Joan attended a Psychiatry meeting at which statistics about suits filed against psychiatrists were given; interestingly, about 82 percent of all suits occurred as a result of a client coming to a first session, not coming back, and the therapist going after the client for payment. In our opinion, it is not worth the trouble to bill a client who has come once and not come back. Other situations may not be worth the trouble either. For example, you may never be paid by a client referred by court mandate or one who has declared bankruptcy. Trying to collect in a bankruptcy may demand more time and energy and therefore money out of your pocket than the settlement you eventually receive, which can end up being only 10 to 20 cents on the dollar.

At some point you may want to consider using a collection agency or going to Small Claims Court. Ralph indicates clearly on his fee contract that his group sometimes uses a collection agency. You need to weigh the costs of going either of these routes with the expected return (leaving aside for the moment the issue of intangible returns). A collection agency usually charges a percentage of whatever it collects, and this percentage varies with the size of the account and your business in general. Small Claims Court is usually for claims ranging up to $1000 or so (depending on local laws); serving the papers usually costs an additional fee, the amount of which depends on whether the papers can be served through the mail or require a process-server. Ralph has been to Small Claims only two or three times.

One time happened to be for a guy who I walked out my back door to his Mercedes. The guy said, "I've been owing you (whatever the amount was) for a long time, eventually I'll get it paid." I was thinking, "They haven't repossessed your car." So we ended up in Small Claims. The hearing officer said, "Are you disputing the services by Dr. Earle? Did he perform those services?" The guy said, "I'm not disputing it at all—I think he did a good job. He was very helpful." The officer said, "Well, pay your bill." Sometimes tough is important. In our case, because we're a group, we have somebody else (in our case, a comptroller, but it could be another therapist) to be tough for us.

Third-party Payment

In its publication *Guide to Private Practice*, the Ridgewood Financial Institute [1984] claims that collection of third-party payments is the most commonly cited practice problem. Third-party payments are those provided by an insurer. The

Institute offers "nine rules for avoiding reimbursement traps" (Reprinted with permission from Ridgewood Financial Institute, 1984, Section 6, pp. 1–4).

1. *Collect your fees directly from patients.* This is [t]he best approach where possible. While you want to do everything feasible to get third parties to pay on claims, you don't want to be left holding the bag if proper reimbursement isn't paid out. At the least, make patients aware immediately that they're responsible for fees, and keep them current on their share of the bill when insurers have a deductible. In general, getting reimbursed directly is a guaranteed path to collection woes and should only be agreed to if absolutely necessary in your type of practice.

2. *Encourage clients to seek reimbursement.* Many don't know about benefits, either because they don't read their plan carefully enough or it's a new feature—many plans have added outpatient mental health care without publicity. Be willing to read over their plan booklets, since some benefits can be tricky—you may need a turndown by Blue Shield, for example, before major medical pays.

3. *Reassure patients about confidentiality.* It's still a very common worry, especially where forms are routinely filed with a company personnel department. For one thing, many personnel offices now bend over backwards on confidentiality; for another, most plans offer the option of direct filing with insurance firms. One company's plan is typical, as explained by its associate director of claims. "When a claim is filed directly, the employer never gets diagnosis information—although it does get a computer printout of the amount paid out to each employee. If you let us know a diagnosis is particularly sensitive," he adds, "we flag it, and that will add an extra measure of safety to our normal nondisclosure rules. Of course, there is an exception—releasing a file to a court under subpoena."

4. *Investigate third parties many patients use.* It can save you time later. Blue Shield plans usually have a local professional relations representative—who'll be glad to sit down and spell out how you can work together more easily. She or he may also try to talk you into signing up to act as a "participating provider," which means you accept the insurance payment as full fee for low-income clients. Most psychotherapists, however, prefer to remain in a nonparticipating status—that way they stay free to apply their own fee schedule as they see fit. With other insurers, you can often increase reimbursements by bird-dogging rejects, writing and calling claims departments until you ferret out their guidelines.

5. *Master the details of government programs.* Buried in the alphabet soup—of agencies, programs, and review bodies—there's a pattern you can figure out, especially important if a significant number of your patients are now eligible. Depending on your location and type of practice, you'll have to gather the key information on claims review procedures of CHAMPUS (Civilian Health and Medical Program of the Uniformed Services), FEHBA (Federal Employees Health Benefit Act), FEP (Federal Employees Plan), Medicare, Medicaid, and the rest of the programs.

6. *Take extra care with claim forms.* Whether you or a secretary files them, it pays to give them a final review before you sign and put them in the mail. Remember, with soaring health insurance claims, review clerks and computers—and often other review procedures—are primed to find any excuse for rejection. Getting all data down accurately and legibly will save everyone endless trouble. Whenever it's possible, try to use the *Standard Health Insurance Claim Form.* This often makes it possible to stock and use one form instead of filing many. Even companies that prefer their own form will often accept it if you send it in.

7. *Review your diagnostic language.* Despite worries about confidentiality, you have to provide an accurate

and understandable diagnosis to get claims paid. There have been exceptions: "We've been paying on claims for 'nervous disorders,' " one insurance official confided to us, "but we're now cracking down hard on that." And many third-party payers are fighting euphemisms: "adult situational reaction" is how one therapist was able to handle claims for schizophrenia until recently. The words of a claims official are typical: "We want as complete a technical diagnosis as the therapist can provide, the same as in his or her own case records. Consistency can help the therapist," he adds, "in case of a malpractice suit." A good source of diagnostic terms is [the current volume of] the *Diagnostic and Statistical Manual of Mental Disorders* from the American Psychiatric Association.

8. *Don't fudge on credentials.* Many plans won't pay non-medical providers, and that tempts some therapists to get physicians [and licensed clinical psychologists] to sign claim forms for them. This not only can lead to legal problems, but also to suits for repayment of fees. It's better to file for reimbursement under your own professional credentials—then fight rejects with evidence of your degrees, license, register listing, etc. You'll often be pleasantly surprised, since firms will often waive their rules. One big insurance company, for example, pays claims from licensed social workers, although that's not provided in their policy and they won't admit it in public. "We know social workers' fees are often lower than those of other therapists," explains a claims official, "so that paying them is a good way to reduce costs." Of course, if work is done under supervision of a physician, make that very clear. And services provided in an "approved clinic" can often qualify for reimbursement, even if the company or agency doesn't consider you an approved service provider.

9. *File claims at the right time.* First mistake: waiting too long to start—one provider waited until a CHAMPUS claim had reached $16,000 before sending it. Few thera-

pists or patients will make that mistake, but they often wait too long. Remember that most contracts disallow claims filed more than a year after service, and while that's often not enforced, late claims usually lead to extra scrutiny. In most cases, it can be a good idea to file the first claim as soon as possible, or if there's a deductible, as soon as that figure has been reached on the account. That will test eligibility for reimbursement and allow time to clear up problems—before bills get so big patients feel overwhelmed if they have to pay themselves. Another mistake is sending the bills too frequently or on an erratic schedule—that means extra work for you. Sending a form in monthly is a practical policy.

The issue of *signing-off* (No. 8)—what is and is not legal—arises frequently in our workshops and warrants elaboration. According to Steven Engelberg, "there is increasing cynicism on the part of insurance carriers about the practices of therapists" (Law and Ethics Workshop, April 20, 1987, Tucson, AZ). Many therapists may have entered into informal contractual relationships with their colleagues solely for the purpose of third-party reimbursement. According to Engelberg, any representation on an insurance form that is not true may not only be misrepresentation (a civil case), but may also be criminal fraud. There have been cases—though not many—in which therapists have been criminally prosecuted because they were providing misleading information on insurance forms. In addition, even though the possibility for criminal liability is remote, the chances for a verdict of civil liability could be much greater and could carry punitive damages with it.

We need to distinguish, however, between committing fraud and positioning yourself to be legally reimbursed. If, for example, you are licensed, you can sign the insurance form, adding your title (certified social worker, for example) and license number. Many times the carrier will pay because you are a licensed provider. It is also perfectly legal to sign the form as the treating provider and have someone else (a psychiatrist, a licensed clinical psychologist, etc.) sign as the supervising provider IF THE RELATIONSHIP BETWEEN YOU IS TRULY SUPERVISORY. A supervisory relationship is defined and determined by the norms of your profession and not by law. Thus, for example, if you are a marriage and family therapist, meeting with your supervisor only once a month and mentioning a case in passing would probably not constitute a supervisory relationship as defined by the practice norms of marriage and family therapy.

Some groups do not identify the treating provider on the claims form, but instead use only the supervisor's/clinical director's name. The role of each person who appears on the form must be delineated. For example, "Dr. Mary Smith, Supervisor" or "Dr. John Smith, Clinical Director, not providing treatment." If you are the supervisor signing off on others' claims, do not claim to be the supervisor or the treating provider unless you actually are, or you could be held liable too. Whatever facts appear on the insurance form must be true.

FINANCIAL PLANNING

In Chapter 3, we discussed the importance of having various professionals available for consulting about clients' needs. In this chapter, we have already mentioned the importance of also having professional consultants for *your* needs. These consultants might include attorneys, accounting and tax professionals, and financial planners and managers. Unless you have the time, aptitude, and inclination to become expert in a number of fields, their services are indispensable. Hiring consultants is not necessarily costly. For example, Steven Engelberg's firm, Keck, Mahin, & Cate, offers a legal consultation plan to AAMFT members that charges a modest flat fee, similar to a retainer, and entitles members to a predetermined number of consulting hours each year.

Cultivating contacts before they are actually needed prevents operating from a crisis mentality. Successful businesses, regardless of field, plan ahead—and planning ahead requires you to extend networking efforts beyond your profession. Advance planning also allows you to interview a variety of professionals to determine with whom you can best work. It is likely you will eventually need access to more than one individual in a given field. For example, the attorney who assists you in setting up your corporation may not be able to do your practice audit or advise you on malpractice issues. Although the following checklist of professional activities may seem obvious, many practitioners have confided in us that when they first began their practices, they were sometimes unsure about whom to see for what. You will notice some overlap in service provided by the various advisors. In general, your decision should be based on the person's expertise relative to your situation and not on the profession itself.

> *Accountant*: basic financial planning (money management, investment opportunities and counseling), tax planning and preparation, establishment of financial records and record-keeping, and general business planning (decisions about expansion, incorporation). The choice of the type of accountant is up to you. You will need a CPA if you are required to produce a certified accounting statement to obtain a bank loan.

> *Attorney*: general legal counsel (litigation, liability, practice audit, contract negotiation), decisions about business structure, malpractice advice, general business and financial planning, initiation of collection procedures, personal legal counsel (wills, estate planning). The legal profession is becoming almost as specialized as the medical profession. Thus, the "general (legal) practitioner" may not be able to serve you as well as a "specialist" on certain issues. Obviously, a malpractice suit may require engaging a specialist in this area.

> *Financial Planners*: money management, investment planning and counseling, brokerage services, retirement and estate planning, insurance, buy/sell agreements. Federally licensed financial planners are designated by the National

Association of Securities Dealers as Registered Investment Advisors or Registered Representatives. The former can advise but cannot carry out the investment transaction; he or she is paid for the consultation; the latter can both advise and complete the investment transaction, however, the registered representative cannot accept money for consultation but is paid a percentage (sales charge or commission) based on the amount of money invested and the type of investment instrument.

Marketing Specialists: market research, brochures, strategies for expansion of practice, positioning, strategic planning for the future. Though most of this book is focused on conducting your own marketing, the marketer can provide you with specialized information, particularly in the area of marketing research, and with feedback on your marketing efforts.

Public Relations and Advertising Specialists: media placement, speaking engagements, interviews, advertising consultation, publicity. In the increasing competition for clients, more practitioners are using the services of these professionals. You need, however, to assess whether using such services enhances or compromises your reputation in your particular community.

INSURANCE

In Chapter 6, we discussed the necessity of protecting yourself with malpractice insurance, but as an independent practitioner you also need to consider other kinds of insurance. If you are just starting an independent practice, your major financial concern is, more than likely, generating enough income to break even. Obviously, the lower you keep your expenses, the more quickly you will reach this point. Thus, many independent practitioners try to scrimp and get by, especially at the beginning, without protecting themselves against various kinds of losses not related to professional practice. We have, we hope, made a case for considering the longer-range implications of scrimping as it relates to the image you project. The same principle holds true about insurance, though for different reasons. Of course, the more profitable a business and the more costly the overhead, the more insurance is needed; however, even fledgling or very small businesses need certain kinds of protection. As your business grows, it is a good idea to re-evaluate regularly your coverage to make sure it is adequate for your current situation. Outdated and inadequate coverage is almost as bad as having none at all.

Five types of insurance coverage need to be considered, according to Sarah E. J. Fajardo, a financial planner with Diversified Financial Planning, a branch office of Boucher, Oemke and Quinn, in Tucson. These include life insurance, overhead expense insurance, disability income insurance, major medical or hospitalization coverage, and casualty/liability insurance. Fajardo summarizes the salient points of each as follows (Personal Communication, March 1989).

Life Insurance

Life insurance is not needed by everyone. Income earners with dependents typically need some type of term life insurance. Life insurance is designed to pay a lump sum to a beneficiary (spouse, child, parent, etc.) who would experience a severe financial loss should the insured die. Life insurance is not designed to make the beneficiary wealthy, but to meet immediate financial obligations and give the survivor time to restructure his or her finances. Life insurance could, for example, pay all debts on the business so it could be sold more easily. Alternatively, if the beneficiary is a child, the payment may support the child until such time as he or she has some other form of support. Life insurance is not an investment, nor should it be used as one. It is simply protection against an unpredictable loss.

Life insurance is purchased to protect dependents against a situation for a specific length of time and can thus be customized to fit your current circumstances. It is also used to protect an investment in a particular item for a specific period of time. This could be a note on equipment, a site, a lease, and so on. You only need cover these financial obligations if and when they occur. When you first open your business, for example, one policy to pay off the business lease or mortgage in the event of your death may be enough. A year later, you may want to add a policy to pay off your home mortgage and bills. Later still, you could add another policy to insure your children's educations. Adding additional policies as you need them lowers the overall cost of insurance.

Overhead Expense Insurance

Overhead expense insurance covers the costs of running a practice. Should the independent practitioner become disabled, the overhead expense coverage pays a monthly amount sufficient to pay the rent or mortgage, utility and phone bills, furniture and equipment lease payments, office staff salaries, malpractice insurance premiums, accountant and attorney fees, property taxes, and other usual and customary monthly expenses. It does not pay the insured's salary.

Overhead expense policies have different waiting periods— once the insured is disabled—before payments begin, and provide different lengths of coverage. The longer the waiting period and/or the shorter period of time covered, the less the policy will cost. That is, a policy with a 90-day waiting period covering expenses for one year will have less expensive premiums than one with a 30-day waiting period with coverage for five years. The practitioner must be sure to set aside enough money to pay all business expenses before the insurance payments begin. This insurance is a tax-deductible business expense.

Disability Income Insurance

Disability income insurance is designed to pay a portion, usually around 66 percent, of the insured's salary should he or she become disabled. The policy will cover a specific salary percentage for a specified period of time; like overhead expense insurance, it also has a waiting period before benefits begin. It will not cover payments past the age of 65. Because most disability income policies do not cover 100 percent of salary, the independent practitioner needs to maintain a savings account to make up the difference in the amount.

Major Medical/Hospitalization Insurance

These days, everyone should have some type of health insurance. Such insurance can provide almost full coverage (including office visits, prescriptions, etc.) to partial coverage that assumes only the costs of major or catastrophic illness. Group health insurance rates are usually less expensive than individual rates. To take advantage of this difference, you as a business owner can purchase insurance for your office staff; other dependents can also be included for an additional cost. Some policies require as few as five employees to constitute a group. If you do not have enough employees, you should also investigate various organizations to which you belong. Sometimes professional organizations, credit unions, or special interest groups (fraternal/sororal organizations, business organizations) offer some type of group major medical to their members.

Many people find health insurance expensive and so elect to take a high deductible, that is, they assume the costs of routine care up to a set amount. Only after that amount has been exceeded, usually in conjunction with a major illness or injury, does the insurance company begin paying. Practitioners currently employed by a company that provides them with health insurance but who are planning to start their own practice may want to see if their coverage is convertible to an individual plan. For example, if you have been a member through a company for a set number of months preceding your going off on your own, some HMOs will allow you to convert your coverage to an individual policy; however, the premiums will be higher.

Casualty and General Liability Insurance

Casualty and general liability insurance are very important whether you work out of your home or in an office. Casualty insurance covers such items as your office furnishings, equipment, files, vehicle, and so on, from loss due to such occurrences as fire, theft, and vandalism. As your practice grows and you acquire more possessions, you may need to update your coverage. General liability insurance protects you against lawsuits resulting from injury to someone on your property or in your office. This coverage may be included in a lease or mortgage agreement. If it is included, you need to check the adequacy of the coverage provided. Again, your coverage may need to be updated periodically as your practice grows and changes. This kind of liability insurance will not protect you against professional liability, that is, malpractice. Professional liability protection is discussed in Chapter 8.

No matter what kind of insurance you are seeking, it is important to obtain quotes from different insurance companies to survey what is available. What is covered, for how long and under what conditions, as well as the cost of the premiums themselves, vary widely. You can gather this information yourself—perhaps with the help of an insurance broker—or you can ask a financial planner who sells more than one company's products to provide you with quotes. Many professionals, independent practitioners included, defer making decisions about purchasing various kinds of insurance, not so much because they cannot afford it, but because they are bewildered by the plethora of options and companies. In fact, much of this bewilderment is the result of unfamiliarity with such simple things as company names and basic forms of coverage. At least in part because they are more familiar with the subject, these same people quite routinely and competently obtain estimates for automobile insurance and update their policies.

PAYROLL TAXES

If your practice includes any employees beyond partners or independent consultants/contractors, your financial planning will require attention to costs incurred by FICA (social security), federal and state withholding taxes, unemployment insurance, worker's compensation, and where applicable, state disability insurance. These are federal and/or state regulated programs; ignoring them is the easiest way to find yourself quickly out of business. The IRS, for example, is unconcerned and unmoved by denial, procrastination, or any other defense, which we as therapists might find perfectly reasonable.

FICA and Withholding Taxes

Connie Bailey, the owner of an accounting firm, notes that (at the time of this writing) FICA charges paid by the employer total 7.51 percent of the employee's gross salary. (A matching amount of FICA is also withheld from the employee's salary.) Federal and state withholding taxes are also based on the employee's gross wage. State percentages vary by state. These taxes are withheld each pay period and remitted at prescribed times based on the amount due.

Federal taxes and FICA are remitted eighth-monthly, monthly, or quarterly, based on the *total* tax liability of a given business. This liability is equal to FICA withheld from employees, the employer's portion of FICA, and the total federal tax withheld. If the taxes due total more than $3,000 before the end of a given month, they are remitted eighth-monthly. (The IRS divides the month into eight segments of from 3–6 days each. If the $3,000 figure is reached during one of these segments, the taxes are due within three working days after the end of the particular segment. Small businesses rarely generate enough taxes to be required to follow this schedule.) If the amount due is less than $3,000, but more than $500, at the end of a month, payment is made monthly. If the tax liability at the end of the first month of a quarter is less than $500, then payment can be carried over to the second month. If the amount owed is still less than $500 at the end of the second month, then the amount can be carried over to the end of the quarter (Personal Communication, March, November, 1989).

Bailey adds that the employer is responsible for calculating, withholding, and forwarding payroll taxes. She strongly suggests that employers maintain a savings account into which they deposit payroll taxes each pay period. She warns employers that the money withheld from employees is "not the employer's to spend. The government will collect these taxes even if the employer's business goes into bankruptcy; in that event, payment is due from the employer's personal funds" (Personal Communication, March 1989).

Self-employed practitioners with no employees obviously do not have to worry about FICA. However, they are subject to self-employment tax, which is a way that the self-employed person pays into social security and becomes eligible for benefits. The tax is calculated as a percentage of net profit. The necessity of paying self-employment tax is independent of the practitioner's income tax liability. Both taxes, however, are subject to the rules governing estimated tax payments. These rules state that if your *net* self-employment income equals or exceeds $400 in a calendar year, you must pay a *quarterly* estimated tax that represents 90 percent of your actual liability for the current year or is equal to or greater than your liability in the preceding year.

Unemployment Insurance

Bonnie McKnight, of the Payroll Tax Control Corp., unravels the web of unemployment insurance and worker's compensation costs by defining the terms and offering cost-containment and compliance strategies. These are useful to the therapist-as-employer and several are useful to the therapist-as-advisor to EAPs and corporations.

Unemployment insurance (UI) is, according to McKnight, "a state-administered program for individuals who are out of work through no fault of their own. Depending upon the particular state regulations and the individual's prior earnings, monetary benefits are available for up to 26 weeks; however, individuals must be actively seeking employment during the time they are receiving benefits'' (Personal Communication, April 1989). The costs of benefits are financed by the employer.

The sole practitioner and group with no employees are not involved in UI. When a for-profit practice does have employees, the state assigns a UI tax rate that the employer is required to pay. The contributions are paid quarterly and range from .01 percent to over 10 percent of the employer's state-taxable payroll, depending on the applicable state formula. Typically, the primary ingredients for determining the assigned annual tax rate are the size of the employer's taxable payroll and the total amount of benefits previously paid to former employees.

Eligibility to draw benefits is contingent on the reason for the loss of employment. Those who qualify are generally unemployed under one of three circumstances: lay-off because of lack of work; termination for reasons other than misconduct; or resignation for compelling reason under state laws.

It is important to note that the employer has the burden of proving misconduct or, in many instances, proving that the employee who resigned did *not* have good cause. Unless employers actively participate in their own cost-control efforts, they will not be able to protect themselves against unwarranted benefit charges and will therefore experience the higher tax rates.

Bonnie McKnight offers the following strategies toward effective cost containment (Personal Communication, April 1989):

1. Generate timely responses to the state agencies on claims from former employers who quit or were terminated for misconduct.
2. Verify all charges with state agencies.
3. Provide documentation on terminations:
   (a) provide and retain written warnings to employees and have them sign these warnings; and
   (b) retain a written account of the final incident that led to the termination.

4. Provide documentation on resignations:
   (a) ALL employees should be given some form of an exit interview;
   (b) a record of that interview should be retained by the employer; and
   (c) retain letters of resignation (however, you cannot require that an employee tender a letter of resignation).

The best protection against claims, McKnight emphasizes, is adherence to the quality personnel practices discussed earlier. She suggests that you maintain personnel records for three years after the person leaves your practice (Personal Communication, April 1989).

Worker's Compensation

McKnight defines worker's compensation as "a state-administered, mandatory provision for compensation to employees for injuries sustained during or arising out of the course of employment" (Personal Communication, April 1989). An example of injuries "arising out of . . ." would be those incurred by an employee who is in an automobile accident while running an errand for the employer.

Again, the employer bears the burden of the claims costs. However, there are several policy practices that can lead to both effective cost control and the creation of a safer workplace. Some of Bonnie McKnight's guidelines include:

1. Following all OSHA (Office of Safety and Health Administration), state, and local safety regulations;
2. Assessing the potential safety problems in your business and creating rules and conditions that will minimize the chance for injury;
3. Posting all rules, issuing copies of them to employees, and retaining a signed acknowledgment of receipt in each employee's personnel file;
4. Establishing a safety incentive program, and acknowledging and rewarding adherence to safety rules;

5. Learning the appropriate action to be taken when an injury is reported and ensuring action is taken;
6. Requiring that employees report all injuries, regardless of how minor they appear to be.

McKnight suggests that independent practitioners include a personnel management consultant in their list of business contacts (Personal Communication, April 1989). These consultants can offer proactive advice on all phases of dealing with employees. They can also help the employer deal with difficulties that might arise. Therapists—whose business is human nature—are at times reluctant to consult personnel experts. While therapeutic and group process skills are most useful in the hiring and retention of employees, a consultant can serve the practitioner in employee relationships in much the same way a clinical supervisor assists with clinical relationships. In addition, they know the laws governing employee relations.

TAX PLANNING

Until you actually start to show a profit in your business, you don't have to worry too much about tax planning. At that point, however, you should begin to develop strategies to minimize your tax liability. You may want to consult an accountant who will be able to offer you tax advice, interpret the financial health of your business based on your financial records, and help keep you in compliance with federal, state and local regulations.

In considering your tax situation, Connie Bailey suggests attention to the following pertinent categories: business deductions for such items as home office and equipment expenses; automobile expenses; business-related travel; educational expenses; entertainment expenses; certain kinds of finance charges; deferment of income and/or payments; and depreciation (Personal Communication, March 1989). Another major area concerns retirement planning. There are many vehicles for building retirement income including pension plans, Keogh plans, and IRAs (individual retirement accounts). The tax advantages or disadvantages change depending on both your particular circumstances and the current tax code. The best sources of information are your accountant, financial planner, attorney, and banker. Numerous books and business magazines discuss this topic in depth.

Vital to tax planning is good record-keeping. First you need to establish what financial information is required for your general business assessment and planning and then develop the most efficient system for recording and organizing that information. Information needs to be recorded regularly. Payroll and accounting services will set up and maintain your records as well as handle the paperwork required for compliance with regulations. Many practitioners find these services time-saving and cost-effective. In fact, Bailey reports, many marginal businesses that might otherwise have floundered have been able to develop successful strategies with a consultant who interpreted the financial information to the business owner (Personal Communications, March 1989).

8/
Your Practice and the Law: Legal Liability and Protection

More than ever, the therapist must retain in the cadre of consultants an attorney with expertise in therapy-practice law. Clients are more likely to litigate than in the past; therapists are more likely to be requested to testify in a trial, have their records subpoenaed, or be held accountable for certain of their clients' behaviors. This chapter highlights some of the most common and confusing legal issues therapists may face. This confusion arises from multiple causes: the courts are attempting to interpret existing laws governing therapeutic practice; professional societies are attempting to formulate guidelines for ethical practice at least in part based on legal decisions; and individual therapists are attempting to apply a general law to specific situations and to balance their interpretation of laws and guidelines with their therapeutic instincts that may conflict with these. The second part of the chapter focuses on ways you can protect yourself against liability even in the midst of ever-changing legal guidelines and decisions.

We cannot emphasize enough the importance of consulting your own attorney about these issues. Our discussion intends to alert you to potential legal difficulties; it is *not* intended as legal advice. These difficulties can be arranged into three broad categories: confidentiality, dual relationships, and negligence. Many of the issues we discuss first arose in a workshop we conducted jointly with Steven Engelberg, whose firm serves as legal counsel to AAMFT. Engelberg underscores the need for therapists to consult their own lawyers because of changing laws, changing interpretations and applications of them, and differences in the laws from state to state.

CONFIDENTIALITY

"Confidentiality is the legal cornerstone of the therapist-client relationship" (Engelberg & Symansky, 1989). For that reason, it is also the area where the therapist is exposed to the greatest liability. The range of confidentiality extends from content of a therapy session to the fact that a given client is being seen. Though no less sacred to them than the priest's "Seal of Confession," therapists are now more frequently asked to violate their mandate of client confidentiality. The reasons are myriad, including court action, potentially dangerous clients, and professional impropriety. The following fictitious case studies illustrate two confidentiality dilemmas.

Janelle is a therapist in independent practice, who specializes in geriatrics. She often is referred clients from an inpatient facility. She had been seeing Carrie for approximately one month. At a recent session, Carrie threatened to kill her sister Louisa who had tried to have her committed. Janelle broke confidentiality by notifying Louisa and the local police of the threat. Carrie did not follow through with her threat, but subsequently sued Janelle for breach of confidentiality. The judge upheld Janelle's duty to warn Louisa and the police and dismissed the suit.

Christopher is a marriage and family therapist in independent practice in a metropolitan area. His client, Jeffrey, was a recovering alcoholic who had been sober for three years. Jeffrey had been involved in an automobile accident and was sued. The plaintiff's attorney petitioned Christopher to testify. The attorney did not know of Jeffrey's history of alcoholism and the defense attorney, obviously, was concerned that he not discover it. At the trial, when questioned by the plaintiff's attorney, Christopher refused to answer any questions relating to Jeffrey, citing his obligation to maintain confidentiality. The judge in this case let Christopher's position stand.

These cases reflect legal decisions about confidentiality. The first indicates that there are cases when the court will uphold a breach of confidentiality. The second illustrates a case when the decision to maintain confidentiality will be supported by the court. Decisions about confidentiality need to be made in light of professional ethics and guidelines as well as an ever-accumulating body of law that varies from state to state. In general there are four circumstances under which confidentiality is overruled: client waiver, court order, mandatory reporting, and duty to warn/protect.

Waivers of Confidentiality

Only a client can waive confidentiality. The therapist must maintain confidentiality unless an exception applies. To waive confidentiality, a patient should sign a release form. (See Appendix II for a sample waiver form.) However, because confidentiality has been waived for one purpose does not mean the privilege is necessarily waived for some other purpose. To protect themselves, therapists should obtain signed releases for each circumstance. Therapists who work with families should follow the AAMFT guideline that each family member who is legally competent must agree to waive confidentiality in order to release information about any individual member. Despite this guideline, attorneys will sometimes insist that the "therapist release those parts of the record that concern only the attorney's client. In such situations we believe that no matter how much pressure the attorney may exert, the appropriate response for the therapist is not to release any information until ordered to do so by a court, even if this forces the therapist to hire a lawyer, or seek the assistance of the other party's lawyer, to institute a proceeding to quash the subpoenas" [Engelberg & Symansky, 1989].

Subpoenas

Because you have received a subpoena does not necessarily mean the therapist-client privilege is waived. Initial subpoenas have nothing to do with whether or not the court has decided to waive privilege; they are merely one party's de-

---

TABLE 5
Witness Pointers*

If you are subpoenaed to be a witnesss—whether as an "expert" witness, without prior agreement, or on your own behalf in a malpractice action—there are a few general guidelines you should follow:

1. Make sure you do not, without authorization, disclose confidential information. A subpoena does not waive the privilege that protects the therapist-client communication. You can testify only if all necessary individuals have waived their privilege or after the judge has ruled that the privilege does not apply to your testimony. If confidentiality of only certain information is waived, either by the court or the client, use extra caution in testifying. Consider whether your response calls for information not covered by the court order or the waiver. Give opposing counsel time to object, or raise the issue yourself and get a direction from the judge.

2. Ask the attorney who has subpoenaed you to review the questions he or she will ask you, and practice "cross-examination" with the attorney. Practicing both direct and cross-examination with your own or your client's attorney is one of the best ways to prepare for your actual testimony. This practice is not cheating; it is a well-accepted way of preparing for trial.

3. Review your records. It is very embarrassing to be contradicted by your own records. Careful review of your records can help prevent this, and refresh your memory so you can give more accurate testimony.

4. If you have had your deposition taken before trial, review it carefully. During cross-examination, many attorneys try to use deposition testimony to impeach the witness, meaning they try to get the witness to say something at the trial that contradicts what he or she said in deposition. As these inconsistencies mount, the jury or the judge may become convinced you lied at the deposition, at the trial, or both. Ask the attorney on your side of the case if you should review other witness depositions. In some cases, review may not be permitted or may not be helpful to the case. In others, it may be a useful tool for preparation.

5. Don't hurry your answers. Give yourself time to listen to the question, think about your answer, and allow objections to be made.

6. Answer the question. This requires careful listening. If you don't hear or understand the question, ask for it to be repeated or reworded.

7. Don't volunteer information. Answer only what has been asked without throwing in extraneous information.

8. Base your testimony only on personal knowledge, not on speculation or guesswork. Don't hesitate to say you don't know or don't recall when either is the case.

9. Be absolutely honest in your answer. Slanting your testimony one way or the other can backfire and ruin an otherwise winnable case.

10. Don't allow yourself to be baited. Some attorneys may try to anger you to make you appear irrational or to disconcert you enough to say something that will hurt your case. Remain calm and courteous even if you are provoked.

TABLE 5
Witness Pointers* (*cont.*)

---

11. Don't be intimidated into changing your answers. If you are sure of your answers, say so.
12. If you are nervous about testifying, going to the courthouse or courtroom before the trial may help. Seeing the courtroom before your testify will help you picture the trial.

Your time on the stand should be less than the time you spend preparing. Don't be surprised if your case is set for trial and rescheduled one or more times. Nor is it uncommon for litigants to settle just prior to a trial. Last minute settlements can be both a relief and disappointment to witnesses.

---

*Reprinted with permission from American Association for Marriage and Family Therapy, 1988c, pp. 3–5.

mand for information. While a therapist must respond to a properly served subpoena, his or her response should assert the client's privilege, unless an exception applies (Engelberg & Symansky, 1989). A subpoena is merely a document directing you to go to a certain place. It may tell you to bring certain records, and if it does, you must bring these records and appear to testify. A subpoena does not necessarily require you to testify but merely to show up. If you are subpoenaed by your client's attorney, your only precaution might be to request that your client sign a waiver. If you receive a subpoena from someone other than your client's attorney, your first obligation is to inform your client that someone is trying to obtain information. You should consult your client's attorney if asked to do so. You may give over the requested information if your client signs a waiver of confidentiality (Engelberg, Law and Ethics Workshop, April 20, 1989, Tucson, AZ). If your client does not waive confidentiality, there are a number of ways, in some part depending on state law, to quash the subpoena, and you should consult your own or your client's attorney about how to do so.

The therapist should alert the client about the ramifications of waiving. For example, your file may contain information about the client that is potentially embarrassing or incriminating. If the client waives confidentiality and calls you as a witness, your file may be examined by the other side, and you are subject to cross-examination about it. If you attempt to hold anything back from that file, you may find yourself in legal trouble. Once confidentiality is waived, the other side has the right to see and use everything.

If you are asked to testify, it is not your job to go to court and shade facts, withhold information, alter your records, or hold back records. If you do any of these, you could be accused of obstructing justice (Engelberg, Law and Ethics Workshop, April 20, 1989). If you are ordered by the judge to testify—and remember this is not the same as an initial subpoena—it is your duty to testify and bring with you all records, if so ordered, and not to mislead, misrepresent, or perjure yourself in any way.

Mandatory Reporting

Under mandatory reporting statutes, states require that therapists break confidentiality at times. These statutes generally concern child abuse and neglect. Every state has child abuse reporting laws, though the laws differ. Some states require that you personally observe evidence of abuse; other states require that you have some knowledge of the abuse. These laws often apply across the board to all types of helping professionals, and there are very stringent criminal penalties for failure to report. For your protection, as well as that of your clients, it is imperative that you find out your state's requirements for mandatory reporting and keep informed about how the laws are interpreted by the courts. Therapists should be aware that failure to comply with mandatory reporting statutes may result in private civil liability as well as state imposed sanctions.

Duty to Warn and Duty to Protect

The law has recognized certain situations where preventing harm supersedes maintaining confidentiality. These laws concern third parties that may be at risk, as well as patients at risk. The specifics of these situations are discussed in this chapter under the heading of Negligence.

DUAL RELATIONSHIPS

Aside from confidentiality issues, the most common cause of a professional liability claim against a therapist concerns *dual relationships* (Engelberg & Symansky 1989). Because of the trust and dependency established in therapy, the law has mandated that clients receive special protection against exploitation by the therapist. Such exploitation may take the form of sexual intimacy between therapists and clients, as well as other forms (see Chapter 7, pp. 141–142 on bartering).

As more attention has been focused on this issue, professional groups are attempting to develop clear guidelines on the subject. Many state statutes governing professional conduct make sexual contact between therapist and client grounds for disciplinary action. Such contact after termination of therapy may also result in malpractice claims and disciplinary proceedings. In addition, *therapeutic deception* is also considered grounds for disciplinary action (American Association for Marriage and Family Therapy, 1988a). Therapeutic deception is defined in California laws as the "representation by a psychotherapist that sexual contact with the psychotherapist is consistent with or part of the patient's or former patient's treatment (American Association for Marriage and Family Therapy, 1988a, p. 3).

Therapists should recognize that some insurance companies will not cover malpractice suits concerning sexual contact. At best, they may cover defense costs. Many insurance carriers take the position that a battery, or wrongful touching, is an act of commission, not one of negligence. It is within the purview of the insurance company to protect the therapist only in cases of negligence. New laws may exacerbate the reluctance of insurance companies to get involved in these cases (American Association of Marriage and Family Therapists, 1988a).

The issue of dual relationships is not just confined to sexual relationships between therapists and patients. There are many questions that remain about what constitutes an appropriate or inappropriate dual relationship. While there may be a case here or a statute there dealing with a specific situation, many of these dual relationship issues have not been addressed systematically by the law. For example, while we might all agree that hiring a current client to be a receptionist in one's office is clearly inappropriate, what about hiring that person some years after termination of therapy? Answers to this kind of question currently come from consensus among therapists in a given community or within a given professional group. These answers will vary from group to group and area to area. We emphasize again the need to educate, and continually re-educate, yourself about the norms in your community and your profession.

NEGLIGENCE

The concept of negligence arose from the notion that, under certain circumstances, a person has a legal duty toward some-one else. If this duty is violated and if an injury results from this violation, then the person who did not carry out his or her duty properly may be guilty of negligence. Negligence actions against physicians usually focus on inappropriate diagnosis or treatment. Negligence claims against a therapist are still fairly rare and, with the exception of claims against psychiatrists for improper medication, tend to allege inaction or noncommunication about certain threats that later resulted in harm to the client or a third party (Engelberg & Symansky, 1989).

Suits brought against therapists generally involve treatment of dangerous patients, specifically with regard to the therapist's *duty to warn* and *duty to protect*.

Duty to Warn

The 1976 Tarasoff case is considered a landmark case because it redefined the therapist's legal responsibility in the treatment of dangerous clients (Engelberg & Symansky, 1989). In the Tarasoff case, a young man in therapy threatened in session to kill his girlfriend. The psychiatrist treating the boy alerted the police about the threat but did not tell the girl or her family. After the police released the boy, he murdered the girl. The parents of the girl sued and won a decision against the treating psychiatrist, who was found negligent for not warning the girl about the threats against her.

The Tarasoff decision is not a national law. In most cases, it is not even a state law. Rather, Tarasoff is a doctrine developed by court cases. As such, it is constantly evolving. Some states have passed or are trying to pass laws to limit and define more specifically what duty a therapist has to warn. These laws will help clarify what have sometimes been conflicting court decisions. In the meantime, however, the trend of the law in general seems to be clearly toward duty to warn (Engelberg, Law and Ethics Workshop, April 20, 1989, Tucson, AZ). Even if you have no Tarasoff-type decision in your state, it would probably be wise to act as if there is some kind of duty to warn. Check your local laws to determine if the court has spelled out guidelines.

If there is a choice between violating confidentiality and protecting a third party from getting killed or injured, court decisions seem to indicate you must err on the side of warning. The problem is, though, if you act too precipitously, you could find yourself involved in a serious lawsuit.

At the time of this writing, criteria for duty to warn remain ambiguous. Some states have passed laws that limit a therapist's civil liability to cases where the patient makes a specific serious threat against an identifiable victim (Engelberg & Symansky, 1989). These laws delineate what response the therapist should make and what actions are legally required of him or her. The law also protects from suit those therapists who have complied with the prescribed responses and actions.

Other states make it necessary for therapists to predict the *foreseeable* victims of a violent patient's behavior. This is a broader requirement that imposes on the therapist the responsibility to predict harm that may come to a potential victim, whether or not the potential victim is specifically named or the threat specifically identified. For example, there was a case in which a patient was released from a mental institution for Mothers' Day. When he returned, the staff saw him spinning his car on the hospital grounds and driving in a manner they all characterized as reckless. Later that evening, the patient refused to take his prescribed medication. Despite this, the doctor released the patient the next day and instructed him to take his medication. Five days later, the patient struck and injured another driver. The court decided that it was foreseeable that the patient would be involved and possibly injure someone in a traffic accident. It did not matter that there was no identifiable victim (American Association for Marriage and Family Therapy, 1989).

Frequently, foreseeability is a major factor in cases involving suicidal or dangerous patients. A physician's or therapist's ability to control a patient's behavior is another important factor. Physicians/psychiatrists in an inpatient hospital setting have much more control over their patients' behavior than therapists treating clients as outpatients. Therefore, physicians in a hospital setting are often subject to a stricter standard of liability than physicians or other professionals in an outpatient setting [American Association of Marriage and Family Therapists, 1989). All therapists, nevertheless, must be cognizant of the laws and their potential liability in treating dangerous or suicidal patients.

Duty to Protect

Unlike duty to warn, which mandates that the therapist consider third parties threatened by patients, duty to protect involves the therapist's responsibility and the limits to his or her legal liability in cases of patients who are dangerous to themselves. Duty to protect is variously known as duty to prevent or duty to commit. This duty is tricky because you are dealing with a suicidal person. Therapists, both for humanitarian and legal reasons, are in danger if they sit by passively and do nothing. If you are unable to initiate a commitment yourself, we think it is imperative to have the patient seen by a psychiatrist or taken to an emergency room immediately. You want to thoroughly document to whom you spoke, what you said, and what ultimately happened. This situation presents what is probably the most compelling reason to have a well-developed network. Ideally, you need to have immediate access to ER personnel, more than one psychiatrist, and law enforcement officers.

As with duty to warn, states interpret laws regulating duty to protect differently. This has resulted in ambiguity of the extent of the therapist's responsibility and liability. In one case (American Association for Marriage and Family Therapy, 1988b), for example, a state court found that in an outpatient setting, duty to protect did not extend so far as to include taking the client into custody. However, this court linked its decision to specific circumstances, in this case an adult patient in the custody of her parents, and left room for another decision under a different set of facts.

As a result of the Tarasoff decision and other cases concerning liability with suicidal and homicidal patients, many therapists have become increasingly conservative in their treatment approaches (Engelberg & Symansky, 1989). To protect themselves from legal liability, some therapists have come to rely on involuntary institutionalization. In our experience, we have found that most therapists try hard to act in their clients' best interests without being overly self-protective. Yet they feel they must balance this desire to do what is best for the client with the pressures they feel from the threat of litigation. It is unrealistic to expect the limits of liability ever to be completely spelled out for every circumstance. Therefore, we reiterate the importance of therapists' keeping in touch with what is happening in the courts, in professional organizations, and in their communities.

LIABILITY PROTECTION

Despite the rise in litigation, a therapist need not practice in fear if he or she applies some common-sense approaches. In general, questions of liability relate to the structure of the practice, with maximum personal liability assumed by those in sole proprietorships, to least exposure for those who are incorporated. The exception is malpractice liability. Though there are no guarantees against susceptibility to a malpractice judgment, practicing in a manner most consistent with the highest standards in the field may deter the possibility of suit. What those standards are can be determined by analyzing information gleaned from a variety of sources. The most obvious source of information and standards is the set of protocols established while the therapist is in training. However, while educational programs do deal with the basics of therapeutic practice, they rarely discuss the specifics of liability. That information is available from discussions with colleagues, professional meetings, continuing education programs, and through the practice audit.

Colleague Discussions, Professional Meetings, and Continuing Education

Once again the maintenance of a network of colleagues and other professional advisors proves necessary. The new independent practitioner can gather information about fees, referral agencies, contact persons within agencies, and standard operating procedures from colleagues. Less official but no less vital information—such as quirks within referral agencies, track record of insurance company claim payments (and the name of the person inside the company who gets things done!), and the status of regulating statutes—is more easily ascertained from colleagues than from any other source.

Professional meetings provide programs on these topics as well as a wealth of contacts and individuals to serve as "sounding boards" for the practitioner. Long before you read about new ideas and issues in a magazine, journal, or book, they are usually being discussed at professional meetings. Additionally, these meetings often feature invited speakers, sometimes from other professions, who are experts on particularly pressing issues. Your access to such people might be much more limited outside the professional meeting venue.

Continuing education classes represent another means by which to gather up-to-date information about practice norms and liability (among a number of other topics). Some professional organizations and/or states mandate a certain amount of continuing education in a given time period. Such required continuing education is minimal at best. Throughout this book, we emphasize the need for independent practitioners to be self-starters. We think such self-starters need to pursue continuing education opportunities aggressively—above and beyond that which is mandated. Continuing education classes allow you to update your skills and knowledge about a variety of theoretical and practical concerns from a "real world" vantage point. In addition, continuing education classes can help you to update yourself on professional organizations' ethics codes. We think it is vitally important not only to be familiar with a code, but also to realize these codes change over time and require regular monitoring. If you take continuing education classes, you will also be in a good position to see gaps in what is being offered, which may present opportunities for you either to "lobby" for a class not currently offered or, depending on your credentials and training, to offer one yourself.

Practice Audits

A practice audit is similar to a financial audit in that it involves a detailed analysis of business and professional practices. The therapist can invite a senior member of the profession to review all business and therapeutic procedures within a given period of time. The consulting colleague evaluates these practices according to the profession's highest standards and ethics and offers criticism. It may be prudent to request that the audit include a written report of the findings and suggestions. The audited therapist should document the steps taken to respond to the criticisms. Good practice mandates obtaining a waiver of confidentiality from each client whose records will be reviewed.

A practice audit with an attorney is also an excellent preventive against lawsuits. As in the collegial audit, the attorney can identify areas of vulnerability and suggest options. (Again, make sure to obtain written waivers of confidentiality if you need to discuss individual cases.) Although it may be costly, the audit can save the practitioner from the devastating losses of a successful lawsuit filed against him or her.

Malpractice Insurance

Declining to purchase malpractice insurance coverage is not the way to save on expenses in your practice. The need for malpractice insurance rises exponentially in partnerships. Sometimes therapists who do some work for or are affiliated with an institution think they do not need malpractice insurance because the institution is covered. You should check to determine the limits of the institution's coverage and whether or not the specific contractual arrangement you have with the institution allows you to be covered. In addition, it is quite common for the institution, the treating therapist, and/or the clinical supervisor to be named in a suit. Therefore, we think to be safe you should have individual malpractice insurance even if you have institutional coverage.

There are different types of malpractice insurance, the two major being *occurrence* and *claims-made* coverage. Medical malpractice liability is unique among various forms of liability because of its long-term nature. The statutes of limitations are usually long for medical claims, and sometimes claims are not made until years after an alleged incidence of malpractice. With occurrence coverage, if your policy is in force on the date an alleged malpractice action took place, you are covered. When the claim is made is not important. This type of malpractice insurance works like other types of insurance. For example, it is similar to auto insurance in that if you were responsible for an auto accident while your car is insured, your auto insurance would cover you, even if you were to subsequently allow your coverage to lapse.

With claims-made coverage, on the other hand, both the date of the alleged occurrence and the date the claim is made must fall within the period for which you are covered. If you terminate coverage, then a claims-made policy will not cover what happened in the past, even though you may have had coverage at the time. In order to protect yourself in this case, you would have to purchase what is commonly referred to as "tail" coverage—as in you buy it to "protect your tail." (The technical term is *reporting endorsement*.) A "tail" covers you for claims made after the termination date of your policy for something that allegedly occurred during your previous coverage (Jim Courtenay, Mutual Insurance Company of Arizona, Personal Communication, May 1989).

Record-keeping

In order to preclude having their records subpoenaed, some therapists choose not to keep any. We believe that this is, at best, irresponsible. Therapists keep different types of records for different purposes. Some therapists will tape post-session reviews that include perceptions, hunches, and reactions that might be misleading were they to be read or heard by others. They then erase the tapes after writing their formal notes. This technique eliminates your susceptibility to having to release, because of court order, any documents other than your formal notes. Taping allows you to ponder the post-session data and document it in a way that triggers the perception or reaction for you, but does not incriminate your client to a potential reader.

At the same time we are advising you to keep accurate and complete records, we also caution against indiscriminate release of these records. This is an issue that plagues health care institutions and independent practitioners alike. (We are not talking here of court ordered or otherwise mandated release of information.) Often unauthorized releases take place because of oversight, sloppiness, or false assumptions on the part of the record-keeper. Unauthorized release of records have resulted in legal judgments against the therapist responsible (American Association for Marriage and Family Therapy, 1989). For example, a state supreme court upheld a patient's claim for unauthorized release of medical records, in part, because an independent psychiatrist—who has been called in by the patient's employer to evaluate the patient's fitness to return to work—was allowed access to the patient's previous medical records even though the patient had never authorized their release. When the psychiatrist had requested the records, no one had thought to question his right to see the records. When faced with a request for records you should consider the identity of the person requesting them, the content of the records, your relationship with the subject of the records, and other people you have seen in therapy with the subject, in order to decide whether or not you have an obligation to reveal or withhold records.

Afterword

As mental health research continues, areas of specialization open up that enable us to reach more people and to serve them more effectively. We have attempted to provide you with guidelines to facilitate your transition from *private* to *independent* practitioner. We suggest that you keep yourself apprised of advances in the field, establish the needs in your community, and create a niche for yourself. Cultivate local resources and become a resource to colleagues. Take charge of building your practice by *plurking* your way to referrals and contracts.

No matter how we define the specifics of a successful practice for ourselves, it seems to us that fundamentally *success* means having the opportunity in our everyday lives to do what we do best. To accept and embrace the idea of independent practice as a lifestyle is to practically guarantee this opportunity. After all, is not *being ourselves* what we all do best?

Appendix I: Assessments

We hope that in the course of reading this book, you have clarified your goals and your role as the prime marketer of your practice. We encourage you to once again reflect on the issues raised in the questionnaires found in Chapters 1 and 2, but do not refer to your earlier responses until you have completed the same assessments at this point.

SELF-ASSESSMENT

1. List two goals in each of the following categories:

Personal _____
_____
_____

Significant Others _____
_____
_____

Professional _____
_____
_____

Spiritual _____
_____
_____

Humanitarian _____
_____
_____

Other _____
_____
_____

2. List two techniques you are currently using to accomplish these goals:

Personal _____
_____
_____

Significant Others _____
_____
_____

Professional _____
_____
_____

Spiritual _____
_____
_____

Humanitarian _____
_____
_____

Other _____
_____
_____

3. Define your current responsibilities to

Self _____
_____
_____

Significant Others _____
_____
_____

Community _____
_____
_____

Other _____
_____
_____

4. What role does your practice play in your ability to reach your goals?

Personal _____
_____
_____

Significant Others _____
_____
_____

Professional _____
_____
_____

Spiritual _____
_____
_____

Humanitarian _____
_____
_____

Other _____
_____
_____

5. What role does your practice play in inhibiting you from reaching your goals?

Personal _____
_____
_____

Significant Others _____
_____
_____

Professional _____
_____
_____

Spiritual _____
_____
_____

Humanitarian _____
_____
_____

Other _____
_____
_____

6. How can you use your professional life to further your goals?

Personal _____
_____
_____

Significant Others _____
_____
_____

Professional _____
_____
_____

Spiritual _____
_____
_____

Humanitarian _____
_____
_____

Other _____
_____
_____

7. How can you overcome the areas in which your practice inhibits you from accomplishing your goals?

Personal _____
_____
_____

Significant Others _____
_____
_____

Professional _____
_____
_____

Spiritual _____
_____
_____

Humanitarian _____
_____
_____

Other _____
_____
_____

8. What personal qualities are required of the independent practitioner?
_____
_____
_____

9. Which of these qualities do you believe you have?
_____
_____
_____

10. How will these qualities assist you in developing your practice?
_____
_____
_____

11. If you believe you need to develop the qualities you have listed that you do not believe you have, how will you compensate?

_____

_____

_____

12. Comments

_____

_____

_____

The following questionnaire will help you clarify your definitions and priorities for personal and business success.

SUCCESS QUESTIONNAIRE

1. *Check any categories that apply and answer accompanying question(s).*

   Success for me includes:

   Community service _____ What kind? _____

   Control of schedule _____ Documented as _____

   Education _____ What kind and level? _____

   Freedom to take time off _____ How much per year? _____

   Money _____ How much per year? _____

   Number of patients _____ How many? _____

   Power _____ Documented as _____

   Prestige _____ Documented as _____

   Publications _____ What kind? How many? _____

   Referrals _____ How many per month? _____

   Requests from colleagues for consultation _____ What kind? How many? _____

   Time for family? _____ How much? _____

   Time for philanthropy? _____ How much? _____

   Requests for speaking engagements _____ From whom? How many? _____

   Other _____

   _____

   _____

2. The three most important items from above are:

   a) _____

        b) _____

        c) _____

3. The most important item from a, b, and c (Number 2 above) is:

_____

4. To achieve Number 3, I would compromise:

Community service _____ What kind? _____

Control of schedule _____ Documented as _____

Education _____ What kind and level? _____

Freedom to take time off _____ How much per year? _____

Money _____ How much per year? _____

Number of patients _____ How many? _____

Power _____ Documented as _____

Prestige _____ Documented as _____

Publications _____ What kind? How many? _____

Referrals _____ How many per month? _____

Requests from colleagues for consultation _____ What kind? How many? _____

Time for family? _____ How much? _____

Time for philanthropy? _____ How much? _____

Requests for speaking engagements _____ From whom? How many? _____

_____

Other _____

_____

5. To achieve Number 3, I would not compromise:

Community service _____ What kind? _____

Control of schedule _____ Documented as _____

Education _____ What kind and level? _____

Freedom to take time off _____ How much per year? _____

Money _____ How much per year? _____

Number of patients _____ How many? _____

Power _____ Documented as _____

Prestige _____ Documented as _____

Publications _____ What kind? How many? _____

Referrals _____ How many per month? _____

Requests from colleagues for consultation _____ What kind? How many? _____

Time for family? _____ How much? _____

Time for philanthropy? _____ How much? _____

Requests for speaking engagements _____ From whom? How many? _____

Other _____

_____

_____

6. The most successful person I know is _____

7. I define that person as successful because _____

_____

8. The person in Numbers 6 and 7 is successful in business? ____
   personally? _____

9. Success for me is more important:

   in business? _____
   personally? _____
   cannot separate the two _____
   I am not really success-oriented _____

10. Others see me as successful. Yes _____ No _____

    because _____

    _____

11. I define success as _____

    _____

    _____

12. I am/will be successful when/because I _____

    _____

    _____

13. When I am successful, it will mean that _____

    _____

    _____

14. To achieve success, I must _____

    _____

    Why? _____

    _____

    How? _____

    _____

    When? _____

    _____

15. I inhibit my success by _____

    _____

Appendix II: Sample Forms

We offer the following forms as examples of the kinds of forms you might find useful in your independent practice. The forms include one to use in tracking referrals; an "Authorization to Release Information" to waive confidentiality; a "Patient-Therapist Agreement" describing fee policies and procedures; an "Application for Payment Plan" for those clients who cannot or do not want to pay at each session; and a combined patient information—fee agreement form that clients fill out before their first session. As we have suggested throughout this book, you should tailor the forms to your particular practice and modify or add to them as your practice grows and changes.

REFERRALS

DATE	CLIENTS NAME	WHO REFERRED	TELEPHONE #	WHO TOOK REFERRAL	REFERRED TO	WHO WAS 1ST VISIT WITH	DATE FIRST VISIT

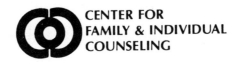

CENTER FOR
FAMILY & INDIVIDUAL
COUNSELING

AUTHORIZATION TO RELEASE INFORMATION

NAME: _____

ADDRESS: _____

CITY: _____ STATE: _____ ZIP: _____

The above named agency is authorized to disclose the following information regarding _____

_____

To:
AGENCY NAME: _____

ADDRESS: _____

CITY:_____ STATE:_____ ZIP:_____

Information to be released (check appropriate box(es):
   ☐ Social History   ☐ Medical History
   ☐ Diagnosis   ☐ Treatment
   ☐ Test Results   ☐ Other
The purpose of this disclosure is (check appropriate box(es):
   ☐ To assist with this individual's evaluation and treatment.
   ☐ Other (specify) _____
I understand that all client information is confidential and my records, with respect to alcohol and drug abuse, are protected under the Federal Confidentiality Regulations and cannot be disclosed without my written consent unless otherwise provided for in the regulations. I understand that I may revoke this authorization at any time, except to the extent that action has already been taken to comply with it. Without my expressed revocation, this authorization will automatically expire:
   ☐ Upon receipt of the information requested;
   ☐ After six months (60 days for alcohol and drug abuse records) from the date of signing;
   ☐ On_____(date supplied by patient); or
   ☐ Under the following conditions: _____
I further acknowledge that the information being released was fully explained to me and this consent is given on my own free will.

_____
(Signature of Patient)

_____
(Date)

_____
(Witness' Signature)

If patient unable to sign, give reason: _____

_____

_____
(Signature of legally authorized representitive)

_____
(Date)

_____
(Relationship to patient)

_____
(Witness' Signature)
A photocopy of this release is valid

PSYCHOLOGICAL COUNSELING SERVICES, LTD.
PATIENT-THERAPIST AGREEMENT

Fees are an important issue to anyone receiving professional services. This sheet was prepared to clarify fee policies.

FEE RATE: The basic fee is $100 per 45 minute session. Longer or shorter sessions are prorated from this basic fee. Fees for psychological testing are based on time spent with the client plus time required for scoring and interpreting test data. Diagnostic/psychological testing reports will not be issued until you have made full payment for these reports.

PHONE CONSULTATION: Our standard prorated fee will be charged for telephone time.

PAYMENT METHOD: Payment is required at the time services are rendered. Payment may be made by check, cash or credit card. Should an account remain unpaid, due to unforeseen circumstances, after thirty (30) days at 1 1/2% (18% per annum) REBILLING AND INTEREST CHARGE shall be added beginning the 31st day until the charges are paid in full. Office visits will not be rescheduled until new payment arrangements are made. These arrangements must be made with our Comptroller. Defaulted accounts may be sent to collection, and if a lawyer is hired to collect the outstanding balance and occurring charges, patient agrees to pay all costs and a reasonable attorney's fee incurred.

MISSED APPOINTMENTS: If you are unable to keep an appointment, please notify the office immediately. If an appointment is cancelled or missed without 24 hours prior notice, you will be billed for the session.

INSURANCE AND THIRD PARTY PAYMENTS: As a general policy, we do not accept insurance assignments and request payment at time of service. If you wish to file with your insurance carrier, the receptionist will give you a bill to send to the insurance company for reimbursement.   There are a few exceptions to this policy (e.g. PPO's). In these particular cases, the patient shall pay all nonallowable, co-payment and deductible charges when services are rendered, and a written change will be added to this agreement to be signed by the patient.

RESPONSIBILITY: The patient (or parent) is considered responsible for payment of professional fees. If we reach written agreement to bill a third party and that third party fails to make timely payments, Comptroller shall notify patient in writing that he/she is responsible for payment. Payment for the full balance will be due within 30 days of the date of that bill. By signing this agreement, patient agrees they have read it carefully and have received a copy of this agreement. Any questions regarding billing, please let therapist know at beginning of session.

_____   _____
Date   Patient/Guardian Signature

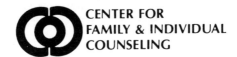

CENTER FOR FAMILY & INDIVIDUAL COUNSELING

APPLICATION FOR PAYMENT PLAN

NAME _____

        Last   First   Middle

ADDRESS_____

        Street   Zip   How Long?

                                                              Own_____Rent_____

If less than 1 year at this address:

Previous address_____

               Address   City   State   Zip

EMPLOYER_____

        Company   Address   Position

If less than 1 year with employer:

Previous employer_____

         Company   Address   Position

Checking Account_____

         Bank   Address   Account#

Savings Account_____

       Bank,   S/L,   Credit Union   Address   Account #

The undersigned attests to the validity of the above information and agrees to pay:

                    $_____ per_____until all amounts owed have been paid in full

I understand that the above payments will not bear interest unless I fail to make a payment when due. In the event I fail to make a payment when due, I agree to pay interest at the rate of one and one-half percent (1-1/2%)per month on the unpaid balance of my account.

I understand that, if I fail to make any payment when due, the entire balance of my account shall be immediately due and payable, without demand.

I understand that I may prepay my account at any time without penalty.

I understand that, if my account is turned over to an attorney for collection, I will pay the reasonable attorney's fee and court costs incurred by this office.

I hereby waive my rights to any notices and/or demands in connection with the delivery, acceptance and default of this Promissory Note.

I understand this Note is payable at 430 N. Tucson Blvd., Tucson, AZ 85716

_____   _____

                 Name   Date

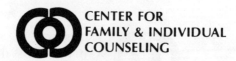

CENTER FOR
FAMILY & INDIVIDUAL
COUNSELING

Mr.
Mrs.
Miss _____

| Patient's Last Name | First Name | Middle |

/   /   /   /

Social Security Number   Date of Birth

Address-Street, Apt.#   City/State   Zip Code   Home Phone

Employed By   Employer's Address   Occupation   Bus. Phone

Spouse's Name   Employed By   Spouse's Occupation

Employer's Address   Bus. Phone

Nearest Relative or friend (not living with patient)   Relationship to patient   Phone

Responsible Party
If patient not responsible for the bill, please indicate who is responsible for the bill:

Name   Address   City/ State   Zip Code

Home Phone   Relationship to Patient   Occupation

Employer   Employer's Address   City/State   Zip Code

Method of Payment: ☐ CASH   ☐ CHECK   ☐ CREDIT CARD (Master Card, Visa) _____ ☐ OTHER

I N S U R A N C E I N F O				
Subscriber's Name	Co., Name & Address	☐Group	☐Individual	
		Group#	Certificate#	
Subscriber's Name	Co., Name & Address	☐Group	☐Individual	
		Group#	Certificate#	
OTHER		MEDICARE		
WORKMAN'S COMPENSATION				
Name of Company	Address of Company		Phone	Date of Injury
			Claim#	

REFERRED BY: _____

FAMILY PHYSICIAN: _____

MEDICATIONS: _____

MARITAL STATUS: Single_____ Married_____ Separated_____ Divorced_____ Widowed_____

   Number of years married_____ Prior Marriages Yes_____ No_____

IF CLIENT IS A STUDENT _____
   School   Attending   Grade   Teacher

PLEASE LIST ALL MEMBERS OF YOUR HOUSEHOLD, INCLUDING YOURSELF, AND THEIR
RELATIONSHIP TO YOU (ONLY PEOPLE LIVING WITH YOU)
   NAME (First and Last)   Birthdate   Relationship

_____

_____

_____

_____

_____

I UNDERSTAND THAT I AM FINANCIALLY RESPONSIBLE FOR THE PAYMENT OF ALL CHARGES
RENDERED TO ME, OR TO ANY MEMBERS OF MY FAMILY, AND THAT PAYMENT IS EXPECTED
AT THE TIME SERVICE IS RENDERED, REGARDLESS OF ANY INSURANCE COVERAGE I MAY
ANTICIPATE. I FURTHER UNDERSTAND THAT TRAVEL TIME FOR ANY SCHOOL, HOME OR
OTHER VISIT THAT MY THERAPIST MAKES AT MY REQUEST WILL BE BILLED ON THE BASIS OF
MY THERAPIST'S REGULAR RATE.

I UNDERSTAND THAT THERE WILL BE A CHARGE FOR APPOINTMENTS NOT CANCELLED 24
HOURS IN ADVANCE, UNLESS WE CAN FILL THE APPOINTED TIME.

I UNDERSTAND THAT, SHOULD ANY LEGAL ACTION BE NECESSARY TO COLLECT ANY
AMOUNTS OWED BY ME, I WILL BE RESPONSIBLE FOR ANY AND ALL COSTS AND ATTORNEY
FEES.

I HAVE READ AND UNDERSTAND THE ABOVE STATEMENTS, AND I HAVE RECEIVED A COPY
OF THIS AGREEMENT.

   Signature _____

   Date _____

Suggested Readings

Bradway, B.M. (1982). *Strategic Marketing: A Handbook for Entrepreneurs and Managers*. Reading, MA: Addison Wesley.

Hofling, C.K. (1981). *Law and Ethics in the Practice of Psychiatry*. New York: Brunner/Mazel.

Levinson, J.C. (1985). *Guerrilla Marketing Attack: New Strategies, Tactics, and Weapons for Winning Big Profits for your Small Business*. Boston: Houghton Mifflin.

McQuown, J.M. (1984). *Inc. Yourself*. New York: Warner Books.

Small Business Administration. *Directory of Business Development Publications, Form SBA 115 A-M*. Superintendent of Documents, U.S. Government Printing Office, Washington, D.C. 20402.

Smith, S.R., & Meyer, R.G. (1987). *Law, Behavior, and Mental Health: Policy and Practice*. New York: New York University Press.

Walfish, S., & Coovert, D.L. (1989). Beginning and maintaining an independent practice: A delphi poll. *Professional Psychology: Research and Practice, 20*, 54–55.

Woody, R.H. (1989). *Mental Health Practice: Modern Marketing, Management, and Legal Strategies*. San Francisco: Jossey-Bass.

References

Adams, J. (1987, January/February). A brave new world for private practice? *The Family Therapy Networker*, pp. 18–25.

Adams, J. (1987, January/February). The alphabet soup. *The Family Therapy Networker*, p. 24.

American Association for Marriage and Family Therapy (1988a). California passes laws on patient/therapist sex. *AAMFT Legal Consultation Plan Newsletter, III* (1), 3–4.

American Association for Marriage and Family Therapy (1988b). Jury gives widow $1.4 million in wrongful death case—Psychiatrist violates duty to protect the public from harm. *AAMFT Legal Consultation Plan Newsletter, III* (2), 3–5.

American Association for Marriage and Family Therapy (1988c). Witness Pointers. *AAMFT Legal Consultation Plan Newsletter, III* (3), 3–5.

American Association for Marriage and Family Therapy (1989). Claim for improper release of records. *AAMFT Legal Consultation Plan Newsletter, V* (1), 8–10.

D'Andrea, R. (1988, April/May). Health plan alphabet soup: A glossary of terms. *Tucson Magazine*, p. 77.

Earle, R., & Crow, R.G. (1989). *Lonely All the Time*. New York: Pocket Books.

Engelberg, S.L., & Symansky, J. (1989, March/April). Ethics and the law. *The Family Therapy Networker*, pp. 30–31.

Farrell, A.D. (1989). Impact of computers on professional practice: A survey of current practices and attitudes. *Professional Psychology: Research and Practice, 20*, 172–178.

Fisher, R., & Ury, W., with Patton, B. (Ed.). (1983). *Getting to Yes: Negotiating Agreement Without Giving In*. New York: Penguin Books. (Boston: Houghton Mifflin, 1981.)

Jarvis-Kirkendall, C., & Kirkendall, J. (1989). *Without Consent: How to Overcome Child Sexual Abuse*. Scottsdale, AZ: Swan Press.

McKnight, B. (1988, Fall). Tips on the promotion of job satisfaction. *Interchange*. Los Angeles: Payroll Tax Control Corporation.

Minars, D. (1987). *Business Start-Ups: The Professional's Guide to Tax and Financial Strategies*. Englewood Cliffs, NJ: Prentice-Hall.

Mitchell, L.S. (1983). *For Women: Managing Your Business*. Washington, D.C.: Small Business Administration.

Ridgewood Financial Institute, Inc. (1984). *Psychotherapy Finances Guide to Private Practice*. Hawthorne, NJ: Ridgewood Financial Institute, Inc.

Schwebel, A., et al. (1989). *A Guide to a Happier Family*. Los Angeles: J.P. Tarcher.

Schwebel, R. (1989). *Saying No Is Not Enough: Raising Children Who Make Wise Decisions About Drugs—A Positive Prevention Guide for Parents*. New York: Newmarket Publishing and Communications.

Warmke, R.F., Palmer, G.D., & Nolan, C.A. (1976). *Marketing in Action* (eighth ed.). Cincinnati, OH: South-Western Publishing.

Index